"This has to be one of the best books of the decade on yoga in general as well as being a 'first' in discussing yoga for men (although women will love it, too). The book has both depth and breadth. It covers the full spectrum of contemporary and classical yoga practices and at the same time delves deeply into these practices with loads of useful information, precautions, references, photographs, instructions and most importantly a realistic and easy to understand treatment of the subject. What I appreciate the most is the straightforward informative approach without the embellishment and dubious information often found in some contemporary yoga texts. Thomas Claire writes in a way that makes the book difficult to put down and regardless of how experienced or inexperienced a man you are in the practice of yoga, it's sure to be helpful. It will be on the required reading list for all of our students."

—Michael Lee, M.A., Founder, Phoenix Rising Yoga Therapy and author of
Phoenix Rising Yoga Therapy–A Bridge from Body to Soul

"*Yoga for Men* is not only an excellent overview of the many schools of the contemporary yoga scene. It gives practical instruction on how to begin and to deepen your practice."

—Richard Freeman, Senior Teacher of Ashtanga Yoga and Director of
the Yoga Workshop in Boulder, Colorado

"*Yoga for Men* is educational and practical. It illustrates the practice of yoga for men of all ages and interests. Thomas Claire has provided men with everything they will ever need to know about this practice and does so in a way that will encourage and support them on their journey."

—Jon Giswold, Author of *Basic Training* and *Beyond Basic Training*

"*Yoga for Men* is a clear and comprehensive study of the yoga traditions which have been embraced by the serious practitioners of our times. This book is a great tool for men to add a deeper dimension to every area of their lives."

—Ravi Singh, Author of *Kundalini Yoga for Body, Mind, and Beyond*

"*Yoga for Men* offers a storehouse of information for men, or anyone, seeking to deepen their understanding and experience of yoga. The book is easily accessible and clearly presented, and most importantly, Thomas Claire holds true to the authentic teachings of yoga. I highly recommend this book."

—Cain Carroll, Author of *Partner Yoga: Making Contact for Physical,
Emotional, and Spiritual Growth*

"*Yoga for Men* provides an excellent analysis of yoga postures for the male body and mind and their energetic usage, as well as giving a good overview of the main types of yoga most popular in the West today and their relevance for the contemporary yoga student."

—David Frawley, Director of the American Institute of Vedic Studies and
author of numerous books, including *Yoga and Ayurveda* and *Yoga for Your Type*

"Stress is one of the most basic factors that impacts a man's physical, mental, and emotional health. Yoga is one of the best ways to deal with stress. Men facing serious medical conditions can use yoga as a way to gain control and hope in their lives to better cope with their conditions. I've observed that my patients who practice yoga have an inner control, without the use of drugs. I'm also amazed at what good muscle tone these patients have, especially in their core abdominal area. In addition to these physical benefits, they have an inner peace that only seems to grow with time. *Yoga for Men* deals with all of these issues and more. It is an excellent resource for any man who wishes to maintain and improve his health and well-being. This book is destined to become a 'bible' it its field."

—John Montana, M.D, New York City, Internist specializing
in men's health issues

YOGA
for
MEN

Postures for Healthy, Stress-Free Living

THOMAS CLAIRE

New Page
BOOKS

YOGA FOR MEN
EDITED AND TYPESET BY KRISTEN PARKES
Cover design by Cheryl Cohan Finbow
Interior photography by Thomas Amador
Printed in the U.S.A. by Book-mart Press

To order this title, please call toll-free 1-800-CAREER-1 (NJ and Canada: 201-848-0310) to order using VISA or MasterCard, or for further information on books from Career Press.

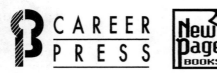

The Career Press, Inc., 3 Tice Road, PO Box 687,
Franklin Lakes, NJ 07417
www.careerpress.com
www.newpagebooks.com

Library of Congress Cataloging-in-Publication Data

Claire, Thomas, 1951 –
  Yoga for men : postures for healthy, stress-free living / by Thomas Claire.
    p. cm.
  Includes bibliographical references (p.) and index.
  ISBN 1-56414-665-0 (paper)
    1. Yoga, Hatha. 2. Men—Health and hygiene. 3. Stress management. 4. Exercise for men. I. Title.

RA781.7.C578 2004
613.7'046'081--dc22

2003058194

IMPORTANT:
PLEASE READ

This book is respectfully dedicated to all seekers of wholeness, balance, and the radiant light of inner peace—men (and women) alike. May your journey of self-exploration bring you ever closer to your own greatest teacher: your inner self.

Author's Note

The practice of yoga is frequently described as both a science and an art. It is, in fact, an entire approach to living that originated thousands of years ago. Yoga has grown, evolved, and branched in many directions in the many centuries that have followed. Because yoga is rooted in such a long and rich tradition of practice, there can be numerous, virtually countless, ways of interpreting and presenting its teachings.

The information in this book is the result of my own exploration and integration of the teachings of yoga—a personal journey that spans more than 30 years. I have attempted to present the many diverse facets of yoga in as complete a manner as possible and in the way in which they are most commonly presented and practiced. I respectfully acknowledge that other practitioners of yoga may view or interpret yoga in their own particular way, and hope that the information contained in this book will be seen and used within the context and intention within which it is presented—to help as many men as possible gain access to the widest and deepest benefits that yoga can offer.

Acknowledgments

Completing a book that covers as many practices and issues as *Yoga for Men* is a daunting task, which could not have been accomplished without the help of many people, most of them sincere practitioners of yoga who volunteered their time and talent to help make this book as reliable, photogenic, and helpful as possible. In addition to the venerated sages of the yoga tradition whose writings and teachings provided the foundational information contained in this book, I would like to acknowledge my indebtedness, in particular, to the following individuals.

To the models of *Yoga for Men*, who came together to show real people doing real yoga: Lola Brooks, Noll Daniel, Mark Donato, Gerrit Geurs, John Howard, Michael Latham, Emily Ranieri, and Alan Rothenberg. Special thanks to Emily for helping to shepherd everyone together; to Alan for providing a safe space for the shoot; and to Noll and Michael for illustrating more eloquently than words, both singly and together, that yoga can be not only skill, but also grace and artistry in action.

To my yoga teachers, who have taught me much. What is best in this book is due to them; what can be improved is of my own doing. Two teachers, in particular, were especially helpful in reviewing the text of *Yoga for Men* for technical assistance: Jon Cassotta and Mark Donato.

To other teachers, practitioners, and authorities in the field of yoga and men's health, who shared their expertise. The following were especially helpful: Prem Anjali; Lila Crutchfield; Richard Faulds; Edward Goldberg, M.D.; Gary Kraftsow; Michael Lee; James Murphy; Swami Ramananda; and Swami Sadasivananda. Many more people, too numerous to cite individually, offered valuable input. You know who you are and I am very grateful to you.

To my friends Clifford Milo and Artour Parmakian, who provided emotional support, a quiet space to craft the final version of this book, and creative and design assistance.

To my agent, Jeanne Fredericks, who believed in this project from the start. And to all the crew at Career Press, who collaborated with and supported *Yoga for Men* from beginning to end—and especially to my editors: Stacey Farkas, Mike Lewis, and Kristen Parkes.

To Thomas Amador, who photographed all the illustrations in *Yoga for Men*. His calm presence helped keep everyone, including myself, centered throughout the shoot—body, soul, and mind. A gifted yoga teacher himself and a wise soul, he used his gifted eye to bring *Yoga for Men* to life. Thank you, Thomas.

Finally, to the many masters of yoga—including T.K.V. Desikachar; Georg Feuerstein, Ph.D.; B.K.S. Iyengar; Jean Klein; Swami Rama; Swamis Sivananda and Vishnu-devananda; and Swami Satchidananda—whose teachings and writings have inspired me and are the whisper behind the words of this book.

CONTENTS

Epigraph

Yoga is skill in action.[1]

—Bhagavad Gita, II-50

Preface

Yoga is a millennia-old body of wisdom that is now exploding in popularity. From urban health clubs to rural retreats, more and more men are experiencing firsthand yoga's power to relax, rejuvenate, and restore balance, harmony, and inner peace.

My own exploration of yoga began more than 30 years ago when I was a young Fulbright teaching assistant pursuing postgraduate studies in Paris. One of my French teaching colleagues invited me to accompany her to a yoga class she was taking to de-stress her life. Curious about this practice called yoga, I accepted her invitation. The class was taught by a young housewife in the somewhat crowded living room of her suburban home. I do not remember much about the actual exercises or other practices we did in that first class. In fact, I slept through much of the hour-and-a-half class despite the intermittent cries that emanated from the upstairs bedroom where children were at play.

I do remember, though, how relaxed and rejuvenated I felt as a result of the class. I was so impressed with yoga's power to balance and to heal that yoga has remained an integral and important part of my life in the decades since then. Upon returning to the United States, I discovered that instruction in yoga is available virtually anywhere.

My life has taken many twists and turns since my student days in Paris. I have earned multiple graduate degrees, and have pursued numerous career paths, including working in publishing, teaching, and wielding the power of a senior financial executive for several of the world's largest and most prestigious companies. And along every step of my way, yoga has been there to support, guide, and encourage me not only to optimize my physical well-being, but also, and perhaps most important, to become who I truly am. Without the courage of self-knowledge that yoga has allowed me to access, I doubt that I could have made any of these changes.

Yoga's great gift is presenting us with the opportunity of uniting body and mind as we delve ever deeper into the mystery of who we are. Yoga is an ongoing process, not a set end point. Yoga can help each of us, wherever we are on our path and whatever our current concerns might be.

The first yoga classes I attended were made up almost completely of women. Over the years, this situation has changed. Many men now are beginning to learn the joys and benefits of yoga. Yoga can support you in reducing stress, maintaining and improving your health and physical fitness, and forming more harmonious and satisfying personal and sexual relationships. It can help you to be more productive in your work and creative pursuits. And last but not least, yoga can help you to attain the qualities of self-acceptance, inner peace, and calm that seem to elude so many men today. My inspiration and goal in writing this book is to help other men understand and profit from the practice of yoga. As with a trusted friend, yoga has served me well, and continues to do so, in my own unfolding journey of health and personal transformation. It is my hope, as well as my conviction, that it can do the same for you.

GETTING STARTED

How to Use This Book

When we begin studying yoga—whether by way of asanas, pranayama, meditation, or studying the Yoga Sutra—*the way in which we learn is the same. The more we progress, the more we become aware of the holistic nature of our being, realizing that we are made of body, breath, mind, and more.... So let us not forget, we can begin practicing yoga from any starting point, but if we are to be complete human beings we must incorporate all aspects of ourselves, and do so step by step.*[1]

—T.K.V. Desikachar

Yoga is hot. Major newspapers and national circulation magazines are devoting more and more feature articles to the booming interest in yoga. Health clubs are capitalizing on the craze for yoga by offering new and innovative classes, and private sessions with trainers and teachers in a dizzying array of styles. Celebrities are signing up personal yoga coaches, and cutting-edge healthcare practitioners, such as Dr. Dean Ornish, M.D., are incorporating yoga into programs designed to help individuals maintain their health and prevent or reverse the onset of disease.

Yoga for Men is intended to answer the questions of every man, or, for that matter, anyone who has interest in this exciting field. This includes those men who may be interested in yoga but confused about where to begin their exploration of it, as well as the millions of men who are already practicing yoga. *Yoga for Men* is for any man who has any interest in his own body and health; any man who has read about the various types of yoga advertised by the local health club, spa, or yoga center; any man with any interest in his own body and min; and any man who may not even have thought about yoga—until now. Although the title of this book is *Yoga for Men*, the subject of yoga is not in and of itself gender-specific. The information contained in this book can also be of valuable assistance to women who are interested in yoga, who may wish to help their male friends, partners, and loved ones benefit from yoga, and who may wish to learn for themselves the many benefits of yoga.

This book is designed to be as simple, clear, complete, and user-friendly as possible. You'll find a wealth of information on yoga, including its history, the philosophy behind it, and detailed presentations of the most widely popular styles of yoga practiced today, including a step-by-step description of a complete yoga practice session that incorporates a full series of postures for healthy, stress-free living.

While this book can be read as a whole from start to finish, each chapter can also be read on its own. *Yoga for Men* is divided into six parts. Following a brief introduction, Part I presents an overview of the principal branches of yoga. Part II takes an in-depth look at the major styles that comprise the hatha yoga tradition, which includes the physical exercises that many people associate with yoga. Part III presents exciting contemporary adaptations of yoga by Western practitioners, mainly American, in addition to some more traditional approaches to this ancient Eastern art. Part IV focuses on how yoga can be used to address specific male needs. Part V addresses the yoga lifestyle, with helpful information for every man regarding a yogic diet, breathing exercises, and meditation techniques. Part VI presents invaluable resource information on how you can find out more about yoga and issues related to men's health, including yoga retreats, books, yoga props, and even some of the most innovative and popular yoga Websites on the Internet. Interspersed throughout the text, you'll find insights from some of America's top male yoga teachers and practitioners on how yoga can be of particular benefit to men. The section titled "A Complete Yoga Practice Session for Men" (pages 112–146) provides illustrations and descriptions to complement your practice. The Afterword provides guidance on how you can put all the pieces of yoga together to custom tailor a practice to meet your own personal needs. A selective general bibliography completes the book, while providing a helpful starting point for continuing your own personal exploration of yoga. Throughout the text, photographs help illustrate the various practices that are being described.

Yoga is first and foremost an experience. According to some venerated sages, the aim of yoga is to allow men to transcend both the body and the mind in a state of original bliss. This feeling-state is a lived experience, not just an intellectual exercise. For this reason, it is essential for each individual man to experiment with yoga in his own way. The presentations of various yoga practices in this book will help you determine which styles or approaches you are most drawn to, and will help you start incorporating them into your life. However, because yoga is a lived experience, it can be very helpful to work with someone who is knowledgeable about yoga and who already has substantial experience incorporating yoga into his or her life.

The best way to learn the practice of yoga is under the guidance of a competent teacher. It is especially helpful for beginning yoga practitioners to study under the supervision of an experienced teacher. Fortunately, the major yoga associations have centers located throughout the United States and the rest of the world. In addition, there are even more qualified private instructors available who are located within convenient reach of virtually any town or city in not only the United States, but also the entire world. *Yoga for Men* contains a detailed listing of resources to help you continue your exploration of this exciting and dynamic field on your own.

Helpful Hints: How to Cultivate Your Own Personal Yoga Practice

Debunking a Few Common Misconceptions About Yoga

Before beginning on our yoga journey, perhaps it's worthwhile to debunk a few commonly held myths about yoga:

- **Yoga is not a religion.** Yoga is a time-venerated system of practices to help you achieve optimal physical, mental, emotional, and spiritual well-being. For those men who are interested in simply improving their physical health, the physical postures of yoga can be of tremendous benefit. For those men seeking deeper self-knowledge, yoga has other tools to aid them.

- **Yoga is for "real" men.** Not only do real men do yoga, but some extremely fit men find the physical demands of some approaches to yoga just as—and sometimes even more—challenging than their traditional fitness activities. Other men appreciate the relaxation and sense of inner peace that yoga can impart. And *all* men can benefit from yoga.

- **You don't have to be in perfect shape to do yoga.** Yoga is not about having the "perfect" body. Yoga is a way to help you achieve the healthiest body and mind you can possibly have. The sooner you begin your practice of yoga, the sooner and the longer you'll be able to reap its many benefits.

How to Choose a Yoga Practice

While many people associate yoga with physical exercise, yoga is more than just a system of stretches and postures. In its largest sense, yoga is a way of life—a comprehensive system of thought that can provide valuable insight into how best to live your life, including not only care of the physical, but also the emotional, mental, and spiritual aspects of your being. This system has evolved over millennia to offer advice and counsel on such varied topics as diet, exercise, breath, meditation, career, right thinking, right work, and much more. Consequently, various branches of yoga have developed that place varying degrees of emphasis on each of these aspects. Throughout this book, you will find detailed information that will enable you to pick and choose what seems most appropriate to your own current needs and desires.

How to Choose a Yoga Teacher

Central to the traditional practice of yoga is the teacher, sometimes known as a *guru* (literally "dispeller of darkness" in Sanskrit). Yoga has largely been preserved and transmitted through an oral tradition. The teacher plays an important role in communicating the wisdom of the yoga tradition, and also serves as an experienced coach to guide the student on the path of yoga. While it is not necessary to have a teacher to study yoga, practicing yoga with a teacher can be an invaluable experience. This does not mean that you have to become a disciple of a touted guru. Simply taking a class at the local health club, community center, or adult education facility can provide you with helpful instruction in the basics of yoga, as well as offer a supportive environment created by like-minded individuals as you begin or continue to explore the world of yoga.

There are many factors to consider in selecting a teacher. The following tips can help you get started in finding the teacher or class that's right for you:

- **Yoga is both an art and a discipline.** As in any healing art, extent of formal training, years of experience, and natural gifts are all important criteria in selecting a teacher.

- **Find out what style of yoga the teacher practices.** Some styles of yoga are gentle and easy, while others can be physically demanding. Match the style of the teacher and the type of yoga he or she teaches to your own style and needs.

- **Check the teacher and/or sponsoring organization's background.** Unlike some other healthcare fields, there is no legal requirement for yoga teachers to be certified or otherwise credentialed. Many teachers seek certification from nationally recognized organizations, while many others do not. Backgrounds vary widely: Find out as much as you can about the specific training of any prospective teacher.

- **Ask for personal recommendations from friends, healthcare providers, fitness specialists, and other individuals whose judgment you value.** Personal recommendation can be the best way of finding a good teacher. However, try to pinpoint what the individual providing the referral likes about the teacher: What your friend values may be different from what you value.

- **Check for professional affiliations.** Many yoga teachers join professional associations, which maintain minimum standards of training and experience, and require members to adhere to a code of ethical conduct.

- **If possible, observe a class in advance or attend a single class before committing to a longer series.** Note the attitude and behavior of the teacher. Is he or she professional? Respectful? Someone with whom you feel you could work well?

- **Look for notices in your local health food store, metaphysical bookstore, or alternative healing center.** You can also find advertisements and listings of yoga teachers in magazines such as *Yoga Journal*, *Yoga International*, and other nationally or locally syndicated publications catering to healthy living. Be aware that these are often paid advertisements and do not necessarily represent the best teachers, or the one who may be right for you.

- **Be aware of any teacher who promises specific results, in particular, dramatic health cures.** A teacher's role is to guide you in the instruction of yoga, not serve as a medical practitioner.

- **Any fees the teacher charges should be within the prevailing range for your geographic area and the background of the teacher.** Expect to pay up to around

$20 for a 60- to 90-minute group class, and around $30 to $100 per hour for private instruction.

How to Make the Most of Your Yoga Practice

While yoga can encompass many practices, most people incorporate the exercise of physical postures into their yoga program. The following hints will help you make the most out of practicing these postures:

■ **Try not to eat at least an hour before and after your session.** Digestion diverts circulation to the internal organs and can draw energy and attention away from your yoga practice. A full stomach might also make certain postures that put pressure on the abdominal area uncomfortable.

■ **Wear loose-fitting, comfortable clothing.** If possible, wear clothing made of all-natural products, as they allow the greatest circulation of energy. Remove contact lenses and any jewelry for optimum comfort. It is preferable to do some poses, such as certain balancing postures, with bare feet to increase surefootedness and sense of balance.

■ **Be as relaxed and comfortable as possible.** If practicing on your own, try to find a space where you will not be interrupted. Turn off the phone or activate your answering machine. Dim the lights. Play relaxing music if you like. Burn some scented incense, light an aromatic candle, or diffuse some pleasing essential oils if that appeals to you.

■ **Make sure that the area where you will be practicing is warm.** Keep a blanket or large towel nearby with which to cover yourself should you become cold during your practice or when lying in any relaxation poses.

■ **Be aware of your body.** Pay particular attention to your breath. Synchronizing your breath with your movements can make your practice even more powerful and effective.

■ **Pay attention to any signals of pain your body might send you during your practice.** Pain is the body's way of warning of potential danger and injury. If you should experience any pain or discomfort during your practice, discontinue the posture in which you feel the pain, and rest.

■ **If you wish to use any props during your practice, assemble them ahead of time and place them nearby.** Props that you might find helpful include non-skid, sticky mats (to aid your balance); wood or foam blocks; straps; belts; and other accessories that might help you achieve a position more easily and with greater stability and comfort. (See Chapter 17 for information on where to acquire such props.)

■ **Be as regular as possible in practice.** Try to find the most convenient time for you to do your practice, and do it regularly at the same time. Some people find early morning the best time to do yoga, while others prefer to do yoga at lunchtime as a midday break, or in the evening for relaxation after a day of work or before going to sleep.

■ Try to perform a yoga session that incorporates a variety of postures that
   provide flow and balance. Tips on different types of postures and how they
   can be sequenced into a yoga session are presented in "A Complete Yoga
   Practice Session for Men."

■ Most important, enjoy! Practitioners of yoga from its earliest days to modern
   times have attested to this ancient art's ability to refresh, rejuvenate, and
   restore.

Important Note: Yoga Is Not a Substitute for Medical Treatment

The practice of yoga can complement your ongoing health maintenance program.
However, it is not intended as a substitute for medical treatment. If you have any particular
medical complaint or concern, or are unsure whether or not you should be practicing yoga
because of a particular physical condition, consult your primary healthcare provider before
embarking on a program of physical yoga exercise. If you experience any pain or discomfort
during a yoga practice session, discontinue your practice and seek appropriate medical
attention.

INTRODUCTION

Yoga arose in the age of the Vedas *and* Upanishads. *It had its beginnings among a healthy, powerful and independent community which had attained a high level of culture. The founders of the tradition were drawn from learned and aristocratic families, from the scholars and warriors. The great prophets of India were kings and princes, leaders of thought and rulers of men. They had the best their time could offer in education and culture, in power and pleasure.*[1]

—Sachindra Kumar Majumdar

What Is Yoga?

The world of yoga is diverse and multifaceted. While most people have probably heard of yoga, many people are somewhat mystified about what it is all about. A common perception is that yoga is a series of physical exercises based on some traditional Asian system. While yoga does indeed embrace a highly refined system of physical postures, it is much more than physical exercise.

The clearest indication of the meaning of yoga is contained in its etymological derivation. The word yoga is derived from the Sanskrit root *yuj*, which literally means "to yoke" (this Sanskrit word is the basis for the words *yoke* and *union* in modern English). Yoga is often described as meaning "union"—a union of the mind and body, and beyond that, of the mind, body, and spirit; union of the individual with all of creation; union of the individual with the life force itself; and unity with the divinity immanent in all of creation.

Yoga originated in India as one of the six classical schools of Hindu philosophy. It is a rich system of practices that aims to help the individual achieve union with the ultimate source of being. Yoga has been described as a therapy, an art, a science, a philosophy, and a discipline. The aim of yoga is no less daunting than to help us discover, through a rich variety of techniques and practices, who we truly are. Physical exercise can be an important tool on our path of self-discovery, for as yoga instructs us, in order for us to find true balance and understanding, it is necessary for us to be as at peace and at home in our bodies as possible.

A Brief Overview of the History of Yoga

The exact date and circumstances of the origin of yoga are unknown. This is because the practice of yoga is so ancient that it is believed to predate the written texts and visual images that depict it. Most scholars trace the origins of yoga to at least 5,000 years ago. Yoga is believed to have originated through the insights and experiments of ancient seekers of wisdom, mystics, and visionaries on the Indian subcontinent. Through intense inner searching, they developed practices that were passed down orally and eventually recorded in a body of text that is considered sacred in the Hindu and other spiritual traditions.

The earliest known writings on yoga are contained in the *Vedas* (Sanskrit for "knowledges"), the most ancient extant Hindu texts. The oldest of these, the *Rig-Veda* ("Knowledge of Praise"), believed by some scholars to date as far back as 3000 B.C.E., contains plentiful references to yoga.[2] Other ancient sacred Hindu writings, including the *Upanishads* ("to sit down close to one's teacher"), helped to codify the oral tradition that formed the basis of yoga.

Some of the earliest and most influential writings on yoga are the *Bhagavad Gita* and the *Yoga Sutras* of Patanjali. The *Bhagavad Gita* ("Lord's Song"), which forms a part of the epic *Mahabharata* ("Great Story of the Bharatas"), is believed to have been composed between the third and fifth centuries B.C.E. Consisting of approximately 700 stanzas, the *Bhagavad Gita* contains crucial instruction by the Hindu god Krishna to the warrior Arjuna on the principles of yoga. The precepts he presents continue to guide the practice of yoga today.

The *Yoga Sutras* (*sutra* means "thread" in Sanskrit and is related to the English word *suture*) is a series of terse aphorisms or maxims that distill the essence of yoga thought. These aphorisms total 195 or 196, depending upon the source text. The *Yoga Sutras* are ascribed to the yoga authority Patanjali, who is believed to have lived between the second and the fifth century C.E. Patanjali is often called the "father of yoga," although his real contribution was to codify existing knowledge of yoga and help provide it a place within classical Hindu philosophy.

One of the most seminal and well-known texts on hatha yoga is the *Hatha Yoga Pradipika* ("Light on the Forceful Yoga" in Sanskrit), written in the 14th century C.E. by Svatmarama Yogin. This text is considered by some scholars to be the most influential text on hatha yoga, the branch of yoga that deals most specifically with the physical discipline of yoga.

Yoga is much more than an archaic codification of information, however. It is a living system of knowledge. Since its inception millennia ago, yoga has continued to grow and evolve. From its origins in prehistoric India, it has been embraced by many systems of thought, including Buddhism, and has become an integral part of the cultures of a number of other countries, including Tibet, Pakistan, and many other Asian civilizations.

Yoga in the West

While many people in the West are only now discovering yoga, knowledge of yoga in the West is not new. In the late 18th century, interest in Sanskrit grew as scholars began to understand the importance and interconnectedness of the Indo-European family of languages. The *Bhagavad Gita* was the first Sanskrit text to be translated into English—in 1785 by the Englishman Charles Wilkins. American statesman Alexander Hamilton visited India, and even gave Sanskrit lessons in Paris, when he was detained there during wartime in 1802.[3]

The transcendentalist movement was influenced by Eastern thought. By the early 19th century, the teachings of the ancient Hindu texts that form the basis of yoga were becoming known to Westerners through the influential work of such intellectuals and writers as Henry David Thoreau and Ralph Waldo Emerson. The work of American and European Romantic artists also resonated with the essence of yoga thought.

What seems to have done the most to bring yoga into popular awareness, however, has been a cross-fertilization of knowledge about India and its sacred traditions that began more recently when a number of master teachers, or gurus, came from India to the West with the professed aim of bringing the ancient teachings of India to Western nations. First among these was Swami Vivekananda (1863–1902), who gained prominence through his presence at the World's Parliament of Religions held in Chicago in 1893. One of the most influential of the Indian gurus was Parmahansa Yogananda (1893–1952), who was sent by his revered master to bring the teachings of yoga to the West in 1920, when he attended a congress of world religions in Boston. In that same year, Parmahansa Yogananda founded the Self-Realization Fellowship, an organization through which he initiated thousands of Westerners into yoga. His *Autobiography of a Yogi* remains one of the most widely read books on yoga throughout the world today. Since these two pioneers, a number of other influential teachers have brought their particular focus on yoga to the West, including, most notably, B.K.S. Iyengar (founder of Iyengar Yoga), Swami Rama (the Himalayan Institute), Swami Satchidananda (Integral Yoga), and Swami Vishnu-devananda (Sivananda Yoga).

The transmission of knowledge of yoga is a two-way avenue, however. Because knowledge about yoga has become more widely available in the West, increasingly large numbers of Americans and Europeans are traveling to India to seek instruction firsthand in the ancient practices of yoga. Ram Dass was one of the first and best-known Westerners to forgo the creature comforts of the West to sit at the feet of a guru in India. He distilled the essence of what he learned in the title of his groundbreaking book *Be Here Now*. Since Ram Dass's pilgrimage, countless other Americans have followed a similar path.

A Note on Yoga Terminology

In referring to yoga, it is common to use the original Sanskrit terms for various concepts and practices, as frequently, equivalent words do not exist in English. *Yoga for Men* adopts the convention of presenting these words in transliterated English, with a literal translation of their meaning generally provided parenthetically. Understanding the etymology of the original Sanskrit word can often be a helpful key to unlocking its meaning in English. Sanskrit terms are generally italicized upon their first occurrence in *Yoga for Men,* with an English translation provided in parentheses. Subsequent uses of the Sanskrit term in the text are not italicized. Because of the complexity of transliterating Sanskrit words into English, Sanskrit words often have variant spellings in English. *Yoga for Men* attempts to use the most frequently encountered spellings.

Several nouns and adjectives are used to describe yoga practitioners and practices that may be new to some readers. A male practitioner of yoga is frequently referred to as a *yogin,* while a female practitioner is referred to as a *yogini.* Alternatively, the word *yogi* refers to any practitioner, regardless of sex. The plural of yogi is *yogis.* The adjective *yogic* does not yet appear in all dictionaries, but is used with increasing frequency as a qualifier to denote that the noun to which it refers has a special yoga connotation. You will find these words used at various times throughout this book.

The Role That Yoga Can Play in Your Health and Wellness Program

The field of yoga is dynamic and exciting. From its original teachings, it has evolved into a rich system of practices that address the harmony and well-being of body, mind, and spirit. It comprises techniques and exercises that can be used to promote clarity of mind, fullness of breath, and soundness of body. From the relaxation benefits of meditation to the improved physical functioning of the musculoskeletal and circulatory systems imparted by the practice of yoga postures, yoga can form an essential part of your individualized health and wellness program. Yoga's reputation for relaxing, rejuvenating, and restoring body and soul are legendary and well earned. Whether you are looking for gentle relaxation or vigorous physical activity, there is a yoga style and practice to fit your needs.

Benefits of Yoga

Prime among yoga's many health benefits is its proven ability to help reduce stress. Experts maintain that up to 80 percent of all illness is caused by stress. The activities and stimuli of contemporary life are constantly triggering what scientists refer to as "the fight or flight" mechanism. This expression refers to the way in which we respond to stress. This response is involuntary, and includes an elevation in heart rate, blood pressure, and the creation of toxic chemicals in the body. Yoga helps to induce the opposite effects, in what Herbert Benson, M.D., termed "the relaxation response" in his groundbreaking book of the same title. Yoga can help to reduce blood pressure, heart rate, and improve circulation to help remove toxic wastes from the body. This may in turn help boost the functioning of the immune system. Yoga is so effective at inducing the relaxation response that many prominent authorities recommend its use for reducing stress and promoting health, including Dean Ornish, M.D., and Jon Kabat-Zinn, Ph.D. Indeed, much to the astonishment of Western scientists, accomplished yogis have demonstrated that they can exert conscious control of heart rate, blood pressure, and even the circulation of the blood.

In addition to its ability to help reduce stress, yoga has many other benefits for a man's health. One of the primary aims of the physical practices of yoga is to help improve the alignment and flexibility of the spine. This is encouraging news for the 70 million Americans who are estimated to seek help for back problems each year. Yoga can help promote overall fitness by both stretching and toning virtually all the muscles in the body. Yoga exercises can help increase range of motion in joints and help protect muscles from being injured during sports and athletic activities. They can also help to lengthen and restore muscles after exercise.

Yoga postures can help improve circulation and eliminate toxic waste substances from the body. They can help promote optimum functioning of the internal organs by helping to massage and tone them. Yoga postures can help open the area of the pelvis and organs of reproduction that are housed there. Yoga practices can help bring increased circulation, muscular control, and awareness to a man's sexual region, thus promoting enhanced sexual enjoyment.

The breathing practices of yoga can help improve lung capacity and posture, and harmonize body and mind. The meditation practices of yoga can help still the mind and bring about greater inner clarity, peace of mind, and self-understanding and acceptance. This can help lead to greater emotional awareness and stability. For those men seeking spiritual enlightenment, yoga has a variety of techniques that can help support and guide you on your path.

Yoga can form a cornerstone of your ongoing health maintenance program. As more and more men are discovering, it is increasingly important for them to take charge of their own physical fitness and healthcare. The physical postures of yoga can offer a refreshing alternative to high-impact cardiovascular and strenuous bodybuilding practices, an especially attractive option for a population that is increasingly aging. Yoga also offers a man the opportunity to become much more aware of his own body. Through the mindfulness and awareness that yoga engenders, a man has the opportunity of listening more carefully to his body so that he might detect pain, discomfort, and other warning signs early enough to take preventative action before illness or disease sets in.

In addition to its overall health benefits, yoga can be of special value to men, in particular, by helping them to contact their inner resources. As many top yoga teachers underscore, today's man is often caught up in the pressures of work and conforming to society's perceived expectations. This can result in a man's armoring himself and losing touch with his inner self. Yoga practice can provide a man with the opportunity to reconnect with himself and to accept himself just as he is—not as he feels he is "supposed" to be. Through a sustained yoga practice, a man can experience the priceless benefits of peace and happiness that can accompany self-awareness and self-acceptance.

Cautions for Yoga

Yoga encompasses a wide variety of practices, from physical postures to meditation. Every man should be able to find a yoga practice suitable to his needs. However, the physical postures of yoga can place specific demands on a man's body. The following are some common, but by no means exhaustive, cautions to consider for anyone when approaching a practice of yoga. Anyone with a history of high blood pressure or any other cardiovascular disorders; glaucoma or other eye problems; recent surgeries or injuries; particular neck, back, or vertebral disk problems; or any joint problems, particularly in the areas of the knees and shoulders, should consult with a physician as some yoga practices may be inadvisable. In addition, for any female readers of this book, special precautions may be appropriate for pregnant or menstruating women. And any individual—man or woman—who has any particular concern should consult with his or her physician before embarking on a practice of yoga.

The Evolving Role of Yoga

Yoga is a lived experience. It is dynamic. It continues to grow and evolve, just as each of us continues to grow and evolve. As more and more people discover for themselves the diverse benefits of yoga, they are adapting yoga to suit specific interests and needs. This is especially true in the West, which has always prized individual creative energy. Yoga is exploding in new directions today as practitioners and devotees continue to find new ways to integrate yoga into their lives. Yoga is being adapted for use by handicapped and disabled persons, by individuals coping with HIV, by senior citizens seeking gentle exercise, and by athletes training for peak performance. Yoga is being merged with journal writing and talk therapy to access ever-deeper levels of the body/mind. It is being combined with dance and movement to enhance creativity, natural expression, and the sheer enjoyment of one's own body in movement. Yoga is being shared with partners for a particularly nurturing practice.

Yoga for Men introduces you to all of these and many more ways in which you can incorporate yoga into your life. The most important aspect of yoga, though, is the actual experience of the practice itself. In this book, you will find all the information and inspiration you need to begin your practice of yoga if you are a novice, or take it to a higher level if you are already somewhat knowledgeable. It is up to you, however, to take the first step in putting that information into practice in your daily life. It is my hope that you will take that first step now: Discover for yourself the joy, peace, and harmony that are the gifts of yoga. They are your birthright.

Suggested Further Resources

The *Bhagavad Gita* is considered by many authorities to be the most influential text ever composed on yoga. Many translations of this important text exist in English. The following versions are especially recommended:

Swami Sivananda, translator, *The Bhagavad Gita, 10th edition* (Divine Life Society, 1995). This translation and commentary were written by one of the most influential teachers of yoga of the 20th century.

Eknath Easwaran, *The Bhagavad Gita for Daily Living* (Niligri Press, 1985). In this three-volume series, a contemporary teacher of yoga comments verse by verse upon this seminal text to show how its ancient wisdom can help guide us today.

The *Yoga Sutras* of Patanjali outline in bare yet clear language the entire system of thought upon which yoga is built. Nearly every major authority on yoga has written commentaries on these sutras that provide great insight into the heart of yoga. Among the best are the following:

Bernard Bouanchaud, *The Essence of Yoga: Reflections on the Yoga Sutras of Patanjali* (Rudra Press, 1997). This book offers a commentary on the aphorisms of Patanjali as well as numerous thought-provoking self-study questions for each aphorism. The book contains insights which the author, a Frenchman, gleaned from studies with yoga master T.K.V. Desikachar in Madras, India.

T.K.V. Desikachar, *The Heart of Yoga: Developing a Personal Practice of Yoga* (Inner Traditions, 1995). T.K.V. Desikachar is the son of Sri Tirumalai Krishnamacharya, one of India's greatest yogis, who taught not only Desikachar but also many other living yoga masters, including B.K.S. Iyengar. This book, which is Desikachar's general introduction to yoga, contains a section providing concise commentaries on each of Patanjali's aphorisms.

Georg Feuerstein, Ph.D., *The Yoga-Sutra of Patanjali* (Inner Traditions, 1985). These commentaries were written by one of the leading authorities on yoga.

Georg Feuerstein, Ph.D., is one of the leading scholars conducting research into yoga and presenting the information contained in the ancient scriptures to a Western audience. He has authored many books, of which the following are particularly recommended:

Georg Feuerstein, Ph.D., *The Shambhala Encyclopedia of Yoga* (Shambhala, 1997). This comprehensive encyclopedia of yoga contains more than 2,000 entries on topics related to yoga.

————, *The Shambhala Guide to Yoga* (Shambhala, 1996). This is an introduction to the principles of yoga that provides particularly valuable information on the historical tradition of yoga and the yogic texts that have helped define it.

————, *The Yoga Tradition* (Hohm Press, 2001). This is one of the most comprehensive books ever written on the history, literature, philosophy, and practice of yoga.

PART I

OVERVIEW
Yoga as a Living Tree

As with a living tree, yoga is a dynamic system comprised of many branches and limbs. In this section, you'll discover what the branches of yoga are so that you'll be well equipped to begin or deepen your journey into yoga.

Chapter 1

THE TREE OF YOGA

Thus, the tree of yoga ... leads us by its practice through layer after layer of our being, till we come to live and experience the ambrosia of the fruit of yoga, which is the sight of the soul.[1]

—B.K.S. Iyengar

Yoga is frequently likened to a tree. Akin to a tree, it is a living, vibrant system, comprised of many branches and limbs. Akin to a tree, it sprouts new growths as it develops and evolves over time. Each of these branches and limbs has its individual name, as well as its own subsystems with their unique names. It is for this reason that yoga can sometimes seem confusing. Anyone interested in yoga soon comes to realize the myriad diversity of these systems of yoga—hatha yoga, power yoga, kundalini yoga, tantric yoga, and Iyengar yoga are just a few of the more frequently encountered terms.

Understanding that yoga has developed over a 5,000-year period and has extended its reach into many cultures and belief systems can help explain why there are so many approaches to yoga. It is important to realize, however, that as a tree, all the branches and limbs of yoga developed from one initial seed: the goal of liberating the self through the union of body, mind, and soul. Virtually each system of yoga represents a path of inquiry that unfolded from a single starting point: responding to the question, "Who am I?" Each of the systems of yoga represents a particular approach to realizing self-understanding and liberation. None of the systems is superior or inferior to any other. Each system or approach merely emphasizes certain aspects of yoga as the path to liberation. These systems do not have to be viewed as mutually exclusive. Each system offers valuable insight.

We have arrived at an exciting time in the development of yoga. As practiced in India for millennia, yoga has frequently entailed detailed study of a particular path of yoga under the tutelage of a venerated teacher, or guru. As the tree of yoga is becoming embraced in the West, it, in turn, is being influenced by and benefiting from the uniquely individual and creative input from the characteristically Western style of thinking. By understanding what each system of yoga teaches and emphasizes, each individual can decide for himself which elements are most appropriate to his needs. He can then create a uniquely personal practice by drawing selectively from the best elements of yoga. Those men who prefer a more methodical, organized approach are also free to follow the teachings of a particular school or teacher in the time-honored tradition of guru study. Your practice of yoga will be your own personal decision.

The following outline of the major branches and limbs of yoga will help demystify the many diverse names you may have heard for systems of yoga. It will help you to get a bird's-eye view of the overall organizational system of yoga without becoming overwhelmed in the intricacies of the details of each. You can then choose, through the remaining chapters in this book, to learn more about a particular style of yoga or practice. Throughout this book, you will also find a wealth of resource information to help you learn more about a particular approach to yoga you might like to explore further.

The Branches of Yoga

While yoga is a diverse system of practice comprised of many approaches to self-realization, many authorities on yoga concur that there are four major branches of yoga that over time have served as a point of origin for developing a practice of yoga. In addition to these four branches, there are several other systems of yoga that have gained widespread interest and attention in building a yoga practice. These might be considered offshoots, or mini-branches, of the main four branches of yoga. The following descriptions will help you understand the four main branches of yoga, with some of their most important offshoots.

The Four Major Branches of Yoga

As most commonly presented, the four major branches of yoga are *bhakti yoga, jnana yoga, karma yoga,* and *raja yoga.* Understanding the nature of each can help you incorporate yoga into your life in the most meaningful way.

Bhakti Yoga: The Yoga of Devotion

Bhakti literally means "devotion" in Sanskrit. Bhakti yoga is known as the yoga of devotion. Following the path of bhakti yoga requires one to surrender oneself completely to a force or power greater than oneself. That power might be a deity, saint, revered teacher, or a quality, such as love. Through the force of opening one's heart with undivided love and devotion to this higher force, one enters the grace of self-realization. Faith, grace, and love are the hallmarks of bhakti yoga. Mahatama Ghandi and the Dalai Lama, with their open hearts and unswerving devotion to serve, are excellent examples of a *bhakta,* the term that describes a practitioner of bhakti yoga.

Jnana Yoga: The Yoga of Knowledge

Jnana literally means "wisdom" or "knowledge" in Sanskrit. Jnana yoga is known as the yoga of wisdom. Of all the branches of yoga, this path requires the greatest concentration of mental activity. *Jnanins* ("knowers"), or practitioners of jnana yoga, seek enlightenment through the power of mental discrimination and inquiry—learning to differentiate the real from the unreal, and the limited personal self from the unlimited infinite self that is the source of all being. Meditation is the most powerful tool used in the practice of jnana yoga.

Karma Yoga: The Yoga of Action

Karma literally means "action" or "cause" in Sanskrit. Karma yoga is known as the yoga of action. Following the path of karma yoga involves seeking liberation through one's actions in the world. Devoting selfless service to others and practicing one's tasks in life—professional, familial, and otherwise—with perfect awareness and mindfulness without regard for success or failure permits the practitioner of karma yoga to achieve enlightenment and self-liberation. Through karma yoga, even simple and routine tasks such as driving a car or mowing the lawn can be acts of yoga practice if they are offered selflessly and to benefit others in an act of service. Many people associate yoga with asceticism and withdrawal from the external world and the company of others. Karma yoga offers those who are interested in pursuing its path a way of practicing yoga actively in the world.

Raja Yoga: The Royal Yoga

Raja means "royal" in Sanskrit. Raja yoga is known as the royal road to yoga, or the yoga of enlightenment. Of all the branches of yoga, raja yoga is probably the best-known approach to yoga in the West. The practitioner of raja yoga follows a carefully prescribed path composed of eight practices, or limbs, known as *ashtanga* ("eight limbs"), to achieve self-realization. These limbs include many of the best-known and most frequently engaged yoga practices, including physical postures, breath control, and concentration. (These practices will be described in much greater detail in the chapters that follow.) Raja yoga is sometimes referred to as classical yoga because the practices that comprise it are detailed in Patanjali's *Yoga Sutras*, one of the earliest extant texts on the practice of yoga.

The four major branches of yoga form the overall umbrella under which all other yoga practices are subdivided. Each branch, however, need not be considered mutually exclusive. Some practices, such as meditation, are common to more than one branch of yoga. A follower of yoga can also engage in practices from more than one branch—a man can open the heart through bhakti yoga, engage the world mindfully and dutifully through karma yoga, seek mental discernment through jnana yoga, and engage in the liberating practices of raja yoga all at the same time. In fact, a devotee who follows the teachings of all the branches of yoga will find in yoga a nearly perfect system leading to right living, thinking, and self-realization.

The Eight Limbs of Yoga

Raja yoga is frequently described as the scientific path to yoga. This is because it lays out in a very clear, simple, and systematic way a series of steps that a practitioner of yoga can follow to achieve enlightenment. These steps, which are detailed in Patanjali's *Yoga Sutras*, form a sort of ladder, each practice building sequentially on the practice that precedes it. The eight limbs, or rungs, of raja yoga, presented from the first to the eighth are as follows:

1. **Yama.** *Yama* means "self-restraint" or "self-control" in Sanskrit. The yamas are a set of ethical practices, somewhat like the commandments of the Old Testament, which form the basis for spiritual development. In order to be liberated, the yoga aspirant first must abstain from engaging in behavior that will be detrimental to his well-being and that of others. Patanjali prescribes five yamas that are to be observed: nonviolence (*ahimsa*); not telling lies, or being truthful (*satya*); not stealing (*asteya*); not wasting one's sexual energy, or literally, demonstrating "brahmic conduct" (*brahmacarya*); and not being greedy (*aparigraha*). By practicing these five yamas, one develops the self-control necessary for the pursuit of the highest goals of yoga.

2. **Niyama.** *Niyama* means restraint in the sense of "discipline" or "moral observance" in Sanskrit. The niyamas are a set of ethical principles by which the practitioner of yoga is advised to conduct his life. Patanjali details five niyamas that are to be practiced: purity (*saucha*), contentment (*santohsa*), asceticism (*tapas*), study (*svadhyaya*), and surrender to a higher power (*Isvara-pranidhana*). Taken together, the niyamas provide a prescription for right living.

3. **Asana.** *Asana* means "seat" or "posture" in Sanskrit. The asanas are a prescribed set of physical postures, or poses, that are meant to purify and steady both the body and mind. For many people, yoga is synonymous with these postures, which form the basis of what is known as hatha yoga, which is derived from the system of raja yoga. The asanas play such an important role in yoga that they have given rise to many approaches to practicing them. Much of the confusion as to what yoga is in the West is caused by these various approaches to executing the physical postures of yoga. Because of the importance that these poses play in yoga and the diversity of ways in which they can be practiced, the first few sections of *Yoga for Men* are devoted to a description of the various styles of yoga that have developed in response to the practice of raja and hatha yoga.

4. **Pranayama.** *Pranayama* means "control (or extension) of the breath" in Sanskrit. The breath (*prana*) is more than just the air we take in and exhale, however. Breath is also synonymous with vital energy, or the life force. Without breath there is no life. Practitioners of yoga believe that it is essential to learn to control the breath in order to still the mind. Consequently, detailed practices have been developed to enhance the flow of breath, or vital life force. These practices include various ways of inhaling, retaining, and expelling the breath. The practice of pranayama is so vital to yoga that you will find a separate section detailing the most frequently practiced of these breathing techniques in Chapter 16.

5. **Pratyahara.** *Pratyahara* means "withdrawal" or "starving the senses" in Sanskrit. The practice of pratyahara entails withdrawing the senses from sensory objects, as in sleep.

6. **Dharana.** *Dharana* means "concentration" in Sanskrit. Once the practitioner of yoga has withdrawn the senses from external objects, he practices

concentration, for instance, by focusing single-pointedly on an object of awareness, such as a mental image or a sound.

7. **Dhyana.** *Dhyana* means "meditation" in Sanskrit. As the practitioner's concentration develops, it deepens into meditation.

8. **Samadhi.** *Samadhi* means "bliss" or "ecstasy" in Sanskrit. Once the aspirant has perfected the preceding steps on the ladder of yoga, he enters into a state sometimes referred to as superconsciousness, in which the individual self merges with the infinite consciousness of the universe. This state of bliss is the ultimate goal of raja yoga.

These eight practices comprise the eight-runged ladder referred to as *ashtanga yoga*. Taken together, they form a kind of guide to developing self-control. The first two sets of practices prescribe how to establish self-discipline over one's conduct and behavior toward others through a system of do's and don'ts of ethical behavior. The next two practices teach how to achieve self-discipline of the physical body. The last four practices provide detailed instruction on how to gain mastery of the senses and mind, leading to self-realization.

Offshoots of the Major Branches of Yoga

There are many paths to choose from, and all the paths are equally valid.[2]

—Swami Rama

While most authorities on yoga generally agree that bhakti, jnana, karma, and raja are the four major branches of yoga, there are several yoga practices, or traditional approaches to yoga, that have gained prominence, and which might be considered offshoots of the major branches of yoga. You may, or may have already, come across the names of some of these offshoots. Being familiar with the following popular terms will help round out your understanding of yoga.

Kundalini Yoga

Kundalini refers to a powerful energy depicted as a serpent (from *kundala*, which means "coiled"). This energy is stored at the base of the spine, where it lies coiled like a snake. This energy is considered feminine. It lies dormant until properly awakened, at which time it rushes upward through the spine to join with the male aspect of consciousness at the crown of the head, where the union of the feminine and masculine aspects of energy leads to self-realization and enlightenment. Practitioners of kundalini yoga employ specific practices to aid the arousal of this energy. The movement of kundalini energy has been described by some as having the force of a streak of lightning.

The awakening of kundalini energy can be one of the steps on the path to enlightenment. For this reason, various practices have been developed over time to help practitioners cultivate the releasing of this energy as a way of attaining enlightenment. These practices can include physical exercises (asanas) and special breathing techniques (pranayama) combined with meditation and recitation of sacred sounds to raise and release the kundalini energy. Kundalini yoga has become so popular in the West that Chapter 7 is devoted to its practice.

Laya Yoga

Laya means "melting," "dissolution," or "absorption" in Sanskrit. Laya yoga is an approach to meditation that uses rites and special practices, such as breathing, to reach a state of total absorption.

Mantra Yoga

Mantra means "thought" or "instrument of thought" in Sanskrit. (It is believed to be related to the same root that gave rise to the words *mental* and *man* in English.) Mantra yoga uses special sounds as instruments to focus and still the mind. The sages of yoga from time immemorial have maintained that the universe was born of vibration, or sound. Therefore, sound occupies a sacred role in yoga. Certain sounds are believed to have sacred powers. One of the most famous of these sounds is the universal, untranslatable *Om.* Because sound is so vital to the principles of yoga practice, Chapter 16 contains a special section on mantras and guidance on how you might begin to practice them.

Tantra Yoga

Tantra means "loom" in Sanskrit. Tantric yoga uses a variety of practices such as external rituals celebrating the divine feminine principle as well as more internal practices such as meditation and mantra recitation to weave the way to enlightenment. Many scholars believe that the practices of tantra are very ancient. According to some, tantra developed as a reaction to classical yoga practices, which traditionally had been reserved exclusively for certain castes of practitioners, especially men.

Tantra is particularly appealing to men who enjoy communing with others. Rather than withdrawing into himself alone, a man can engage with others in order to achieve liberation. This union can entail sexual union. As a result of this fact, tantric yoga is sometimes mistakenly understood to apply only to sexual practices. Tantra, however, involves a much wider range of rituals that are practiced in a sacred, ceremonial way to imbue them with the power of transformation and self-realization. When tantric practices include sexual acts, these acts are engaged in as a means of achieving self-realization. Kundalini yoga draws on some of the practices that form part of tantra yoga.

Hatha Yoga

Hatha literally means "violence" or "force" in Sanskrit. Hatha yoga is frequently referred to as the "forceful yoga." It generally refers to the practice of the physical postures, or asanas, of yoga. To many people, yoga is synonymous with the practice of these physical postures. A variety of approaches to executing these postures has developed over time; consequently, various approaches to hatha yoga have developed. The following chapters will help you better understand the most important approaches to hatha yoga.

For Further Information

Becoming familiar with the branches and limbs of the tree of yoga is the first and most important step in demystifying yoga. Now that you understand the broad way in which the system of yoga is organized, you can pursue whichever aspect of it you wish. The chapters that immediately follow will introduce you to particular approaches to hatha yoga. These and subsequent sections provide information on specific yoga practices and techniques, such as physical postures, breathing exercises, mantra recitation, and meditation, so that you can begin to practice yoga yourself as you feel ready.

If you should have a particular interest in any one of the branches or approaches to yoga, you will find helpful resources on where to gather further information in each of the individual chapters, as well as in Chapter 17 and the Bibliography.

Suggested Further Resources

If you would like to learn more about the various paths of yoga, the following books are highly recommended:

Sri Swami Rama, *Choosing a Path: Intellect, Action, Devotion, Meditation, Fusion, Primal Force, Tantra* (Himalayan Institute, 1982). This is an informative guide to the major paths of yoga by one of the most famous Indian swamis to have come to the West.

Swami Vivekananda, *Jnana-Yoga, Karma-Yoga and Bhakti-Yoga*, and *Raja-Yoga* (Ramakrishna-Vivekananda Center, 1955). This series of three small books provides insightful commentary on the four principal branches of yoga.

PART II

HATHA YOGA

The Main Traditions

Hatha yoga means literally the "forceful yoga." As its name implies, this approach to yoga emphasizes the vitality and life force of the physical body. Hatha yoga is undoubtedly the most well known, popular, and frequently practiced style of yoga in the West. It places great emphasis on purifying the body through a variety of means that include physical exercise, cleansing rites, and specific breathing techniques. These practices not only strengthen the body through the force of exercise, they can also help you to expand your own personal force, or store of energy, through their vitalizing effects.

One of the most influential and widely read texts on hatha yoga is the *Hatha Yoga Pradipika*, written in the 14th century C.E. In this seminal manual, the author describes 16 physical postures as well as a variety of cleansing and breathing practices and what are known as locks and seals to control the flow of energy within the body.[1]

In its emphasis on physical postures, or asanas, hatha yoga is often considered one of the steps on the eight-limbed path of yoga, which forms an important part of classical, or raja, yoga. However, it is important to bear in mind that emphasis is placed on making the body as whole and complete as possible in order to achieve the ultimate goal of liberation. Practitioners of hatha yoga believe that in order to achieve the fullest unfoldment of our minds and spirits, we must do our utmost to have a body that is at ease and free of disease. Hatha yoga is thus a way of balancing or harmonizing body and mind. This intent is highlighted in the esoteric interpretation sometimes accorded to the word hatha. According to some practitioners, the word *hatha* is comprised of two syllables that stand for the sun (*ha*) and the moon (*tha*), implying a deep union of the body and the mind and of the masculine and feminine energies within each individual—man and woman alike. Thus, the word hatha reminds us that at heart, yoga is a search for underlying unity and wholeness.

41

Hatha yoga practitioners see the body as a wonderful vehicle for self-realization. For without a body, we would not be alive today, and thus incapable of seeking the path of transformation. Hatha yoga urges a man to respect his body as a temple of the divine spirit of the universe. The practice of hatha yoga is thus an opportunity of honoring your own inner divinity.

Hatha yoga has become so popular, particularly in the last few decades, that there are now many styles for practicing it. Surprisingly, however, most of the styles of hatha yoga that are practiced today trace their roots to a handful of yoga teachers, who traveled from India to the West in the 1960s and 1970s to train practitioners here in their particular approach to yoga; or to a small number of Westerners who traveled to India during the same time period to train as teachers with a few celebrated masters.

The teachers of the 60s and 70s differed in their approach to presenting yoga from the gurus who had preceded them. The earliest teachers of yoga who traveled to the West in the late 19th and early 20th centuries emphasized the traditional sacred texts and metaphysical aspects of yoga. The newer generation of teachers, while revering all aspects of the yoga tradition, also incorporated much more of the physical exercise aspect of yoga into their teaching. Their approaches to yoga appealed to Western practitioners, and, consequently, much of the yoga that has developed in the United States has focused on the physical postures of hatha yoga.

The following chapters will introduce you to the main approaches to hatha yoga that have helped to define hatha practice in the West. Because there are now so many styles of yoga available, the choice of a practice can seem overwhelming. These chapters will introduce you to the main styles of hatha yoga so that you can be better informed as you undertake your own practice of yoga.

Each of the main styles of hatha yoga is generally named after the individual who first introduced or was influential in the teachings of that style, such as Iyengar Yoga and Sivananda Yoga; the institute that was founded based on their teachings, such as yoga taught at the Himalayan Institute and Integral Yoga; or for a prominent element or focal point of the approach, such as Ashtanga Yoga and kundalini yoga.

Nearly all the various styles of hatha yoga have as their base a common repertoire of physical postures and practices, which have evolved over the centuries. The emphasis on how to perform these practices can differ widely from one style of yoga to another, however. Understanding the differences among these styles can help you choose the style of hatha yoga that is right for you. The following chapters describe the major styles of hatha yoga that you are likely to encounter in your exploration of yoga today. As you read these chapters, please bear in mind that the approaches to yoga presented are grouped together under hatha yoga for convenience. In addition to instruction in the physical postures of yoga, most of these approaches can also help you incorporate a full range of yogic practices into your life.

Chapter 2

HIMALAYAN INSTITUTE OF YOGA SCIENCE AND PHILOSOPHY

Swami Rama's Scientific Approach to Training the Mind Through the Body

You are a citizen of two worlds—the inner and outer. There should be a bridge between these two worlds.[1]

—Swami Rama

What Is the Himalayan Institute's Approach to Yoga?

The Himalayan Institute of Yoga Science and Philosophy (Himalayan Institute) teaches a holistic yoga that aims to provide a bridge between body and mind. The Himalayan Institute, founded in 1971 by Sri Swami Rama (1925–1996), is a nonprofit organization dedicated to helping people grow physically, mentally, and spiritually by combining the best of the knowledge from both East and West. The Institute's international headquarters is located in Honesdale, Pennsylvania. It offers programs in yoga through branch and affiliated centers throughout the United States and the rest of the world. The Himalayan Institute's approach to yoga utilizes the traditional practices of raja yoga to unify body, mind, and soul.

The Origins of the Himalayan Institute's Teachings on Yoga

The founding and inspirational force behind the Himalayan Institute is Swami Rama and the unbroken lineage of sages in his tradition. Swami Rama was born in North India, and was raised in the tradition of the cave monasteries of the Himalayan mountains. For more than

> The Himalayan Institute approach to yoga is noted for its practical and pragmatic approach. The Institute was founded more than 30 years ago by Swami Rama, and is guided today by Swami Rama's successor and spiritual head of the Institute, Pandit Rajmani Tigunait, Ph.D. The Himalayan Institute remains true to its original mission: to link East and West, spirituality and science, and ancient wisdom and modern technology. In fulfilling its mission, the Himalayan Institute can help every man develop a healthy body, a clear mind, and a joyful spirit, bringing a qualitative change within and without.

four decades he traveled widely, studying at the feet of sages throughout India, Tibet, and Pakistan. He complemented his study of traditional Eastern practices with studies in Western psychology and philosophy at Western universities, including Oxford University in England. In the 1960s, Swami Rama was sent by his master to bring the teachings of yoga to the West, with this pithy message: "Inner strength, cheerfulness, and selfless service are the basic principles of life. It is immaterial whether one lives in the East or West. A human being should be a human being first. Be spontaneous. And let yourself become the instrument to teach pure spirituality without any religion and culture."[2]

Swami Rama arrived in the United States in 1969. He quickly gained recognition in his role as a research consultant to the Menninger Foundation in Topeka, Kansas. He amazed the scientific community by demonstrating that he could control the functioning of his autonomic nervous system and brain. At the Menninger Foundation, Swami Rama demonstrated that it was possible to stop the heart while remaining fully lucid.[3] The results of these experiments revolutionized the way in which the medical community views the functioning of the human being and serve as the basis for the now widespread knowledge about so-called "yogic powers." Two books have been written on his work at the Menninger Foundation: *Swami* (Himalayan Institute) by Doug Boyd and *Beyond Biofeedback* (Rinella Editorial Services) by Alyce Green.

The Himalayan Institute and its many branch locations offer a wide range of programs relating to yoga principles. Swami Rama's dedication to making the principles of yoga a concrete reality is reflected in his establishment of the Himalayan Institute Charitable Hospital in the foothills of the Himalayas. This 500-bed, modern medical facility is the result of the selfless service that was the hallmark of his life and a pillar of yoga. It provides up-to-date medical treatments to the poor.

The spiritual head of the Himalayan Institute, Pandit Rajmani Tigunait, Ph.D., is the successor of Swami Rama of the Himalayas. Pandit Tigunait walks in the footsteps of his master—he writes, teaches, guides, and administers the work and mission of the Himalayan Institute. This mission includes Sacred Link, a project launched by Pandit Tigunait in fall 2001. The mission of Sacred Link is to bring forward thousands of years of cumulative knowledge embodied in the spiritual heritage of people of different faiths, cultures, and ethnic groups.

The Theory Underlying the Himalayan Institute

The approach to yoga taught at the Himalayan Institute is based on the teachings and practices presented by Swami Rama and the 5,000 year–old tradition from which he came.

These teachings form the foundation for the classes and programs that are presented by the Himalayan Institute today under the leadership of Pandit Rajmani Tigunait.

Swami Rama described his approach to yoga as a holistic path. He presented the teachings of yoga in three levels. All levels reflect the yogic belief that body, mind, and spirit are interconnected.

The first level of teaching at the Himalayan Institute reflects the practices of traditional yoga texts and teachings. The *Yoga Sutras* of Patanjali form the main text for these practices. This level emphasizes the eight limbs of raja yoga. Hatha yoga, pranayama, concentration, meditation, selfless service, and the principles of diet and nutrition are all important on this first level. These practices form approximately 90 percent of Swami Rama's teachings.

The second level of Swami Rama's teachings draws its inspiration from the ancient sacred teachings of the *Upanishads*. These texts emphasize the divinity that resides within each man. Realization of this sacred truth leads one to love and embrace all of humanity. As Swami Rama said, "Before we attempt to experience God we must connect ourselves with other human hearts. You are already divine. To experience that, first you have to become human. The magnetism of the human within will pull God toward us, and the divinity within us will awaken spontaneously. This results in the union of the individual self with the Supreme Self."[4]

The third and highest level of Swami Rama's teachings was imparted through silence. This level of teaching confirmed what the student had already learned and experienced. At this level of understanding, the individual self merges into union with the infinite in what is known as *Saundaryalahari*—"The Wave of Beauty and Bliss."

While Swami Rama's teachings are founded on a wide range of ancient metaphysical knowledge, the hallmark of the Himalayan Institute is its practicality. Swami Rama believed that the surest route to self-realization is the path of selfless service, a path that the Himalayan Institute continues to encourage today.

The Himalayan Institute: The Style

Swami Rama taught a complete and systematic approach to guide practitioners to their inner selves. Within this system, hatha yoga is used as a means of training the mind through the body.

The hatha yoga aspect of the Himalayan Institute is most commonly practiced in a class setting or in individual instruction. In either case, teachers of Himalayan Institute Yoga are certified by the Himalayan Institute Teachers Association. Individual instruction by certified Himalayan Institute yoga teachers is also available. Hatha yoga at the Himalayan Institute is comprised of several levels of practice—Gentle, Beginning, Intermediate, and Advanced. While teachers are trained to accommodate all levels of students within one class format, they usually hold separate classes for each level. Classes follow a similar structure, which is composed of a set group of postures that incorporate a balanced set of all the major yoga postures designed for maximum benefit.

Himalayan Institute hatha yoga classes emphasize inner awareness and control of the breath. They also emphasize proper relaxation practices. In addition to classes in hatha yoga, the Himalayan Institute offers courses in meditation, breath control, diet, stress-reduction, and exploration of sacred scriptures.

Because of their very practical approach, Himalayan Institute teachings can be especially effective at reducing stress. At the Honesdale campus, its international headquarters, a number of research projects are currently underway to help assess the benefits of yoga in stress-reduction and in helping a variety of illnesses. The Himalayan Institute is at the cutting edge of providing treatment and instruction in a variety of alternative healing practices, including homeopathy and ayurveda. It provides medical evaluations and treatments at its Honesdale headquarters, as well as at some of its branch locations.

It was Swami Rama's goal to bridge East and West, mind and body. The Himalayan Institute presents a set of concrete, practical tools to accomplish this end. It holds special appeal for men looking for a practical and systematic approach to yoga.

In keeping with its comprehensive, systematic approach to yoga, the Himalayan Institute has developed a program of yoga to suit nearly any man's needs and abilities. For those individuals who are stiff, out of shape, sick, or weak, the Himalayan Institute has an entire series of joint and gland exercises. These exercises are designed to loosen the joints, stimulate circulation, and tonify the glands. The asanas that are practiced in hatha yoga classes can be modified to suit individual needs.

Background and Training of Practitioners

Training and certification at the Himalayan Institute is provided through the Hatha Yoga Teacher Certification Program. The basic training program is comprised of a combination of ongoing personal practice of hatha yoga, training in meditation, home study, a three-week intensive teacher training course conducted at sites throughout the United States as well as in India, practice and evaluation of teaching, a series of written assignments, and examinations. Home study courses focus on essential yoga philosophy, asana practice, science of breath, meditation, anatomy for yoga, and diet and nutrition. Candidates for admission to this teacher training program must have actively practiced hatha yoga for at least two years prior to application for training, including attendance at beginning and intermediate classes and regular daily practice of hatha yoga. Certification of teachers is valid for three years subject to a teacher's meeting certain minimum requirements of teaching, study, and personal practice. In addition to its basic teacher training course, the Institute has recently introduced an Advanced Teacher's Training Program, offered in Allahabad, India. There are currently more than 1,000 certified teachers trained by the Himalayan Institute worldwide.

For Further Information

The Himalayan Institute is located on a 400-acre campus in the rolling hills of the Pocono Mountains in the northeastern Pennsylvania town of Honesdale. It offers a wide range of programs, classes, and seminars ranging from weekends to a week or longer at its Honesdale campus, as well as at its branches and affiliated centers throughout the United States and the rest of the world. These include courses on hatha yoga, meditation, breath control, diet and many other practices related to health and well-being. The international headquarters in Honesdale offers residential programs in self-transformation that allow individuals the opportunity to spend extended periods of time living and working within a yogic community.

The Himalayan Institute publishes a bi-monthly journal titled *Yoga International*, which is one of the leading professional yoga publications. In addition, the Himalayan Institute Press publishes a wide variety of books and tapes on yoga. The Institute also sells various supplies and products to enhance the practice of yoga through its online and mail-order retail stores.

For further information on the Himalayan Institute, its programs and services, or catalog of its products, contact:

Himalayan Institute

RR1 Box 1127

Honesdale, PA 18431-9706

Tel: (800) 822-4547 or (570) 253-5551

Fax: (570) 253-9078

Website: *www.himalayaninstitute.org*

E-mail: info@himalayaninstitute.org (for Himalayan Institute in general)

Hibooks@himalyaninstitute.org (for information on Himalayan Institute books and other products)

To locate a certified Himalayan Institute yoga teacher in your area, or for more information on the Teacher Certification Program, call (570) 253–5551, ext. 1251.

The Himalayan Institute maintains one of the richest Websites on yoga at its principal Web address of *www.himalayaninstitute.org*. Its Website presents articles from the current issue of *Yoga International* magazine, as well as numerous archived articles from past issues on topics as wide-ranging as asana practice, ayurveda, health, meditation, spirituality, and tantra. It presents an "Asana of the Month" in addition to various archived discussions and instructions on a diverse group of asanas. Its *Quarterly Guide to Programs* and *Yoga Teachers Guide* are also available online. Through the "Find a Teacher" searchable database of its *Yoga Teachers Guide*, you can find a yoga teacher near you by entering your city or United States zip code. Information on the site is available in Spanish as well as an English language version.

Suggested Further Resources

The Himalayan Institute operates a publishing arm that is one of the foremost publishers of books on yoga. Swami Rama wrote more than 30 books, and many other authorities on yoga that are affiliated with the Himalayan Institute have written books or produced audiotapes that are published by the Institute. For complete information on the titles that are available, contact the Himalayan Institute. The Himalayan Institute also operates a bookstore, East West Books in New York City, which stocks not only Himalayan Institute books, but also one of the widest selections of books on yoga, spirituality, health, and healing available. It publishes a catalog of the books it offers. Both the catalog and books are available by mail. For further information, see "Mail-Order Book Companies" on page 231.

Among the many books published by the Himalayan Institute, the following are of special interest:

Sandra Anderson and Rolf Sovik, Psy.D., *Yoga: Mastering the Basics* (Himalayan Institute Press, 2002). A comprehensive and practical illustrated guide to the essential elements of yoga, this book covers all aspects of practice: postures, breath training, relaxation, meditation, lifestyle, and fundamental philosophy. This is one of the best overall introductions to yoga available.

Rudolph M. Ballentine, M.D., editor, *The Theory and Practice of Meditation*, 2nd edition (Himalayan Institute Press, 1986). This collection of essays by senior teachers of the Himalayan Institute is an excellent introduction to meditation. This book addresses such issues as the nature of meditation and obstacles to meditation, and provides instruction on how to begin a practice of meditation.

Pandit Rajmani Tigunait, Ph.D., *At the Eleventh Hour: The Biography of Swami Rama* (Himalayan Institute Press, 2001). A heartfelt and inspirational account of the life of Swami Rama, by Swami Rama's student and successor as spiritual head of the Himalayan International Institute.

Swami Rama, Rudolph Ballentine, M.D., and Alan Hymes, M.D., *Science of Breath: A Practical Guide* (Himalayan Institute Press, 1979). This book, which is the collaborative effort of an Eastern spiritual adept and Western medical practitioners, is a useful introduction to the science of breath control, and explores how the breath can be a bridge connecting body, mind, and soul.

Swami Rama and Swami Ajaya, *Creative Use of Emotion* (Himalayan Institute Press, 1976). Because of its ability to tap deep into the unconscious, yoga can play an important role in helping individuals to get more in touch with their emotions and psychological well-being. This book, which teams an Eastern spiritual teacher with a Western psychologist, explores the development of consciousness and its implications for emotionalism.

Nishit Patel on yoga for men:

"I believe that yoga can be especially beneficial for men by helping them to improve their level of physical fitness, and also their breathing. Traditionally, throughout the ages, the practice of yoga was reserved almost exclusively for men. To study yoga required that one go outside of the home, to study asana or meditation with a teacher. Men were allowed to do this, but women traditionally stayed at home.

"This does not mean that there were not many great women saints in India. Indeed, some of the greatest saints in India were women. Women followed the path of bhakti yoga, or complete surrender and devotion to their husbands and family duties. Through their one-pointed selfless service, such women attained liberation."

—Nishit Patel, Director of the Himalayan Institute in New York City

Chapter 3

INTEGRAL YOGA

Sri Swami Satchidananda's Meditation for the Body

Integral Yoga: Peaceful, Easeful, Useful.

—Sri Swami Satchidananda

What Is Integral Yoga?

Integral Yoga, as its name implies, is a system of yoga that aims to integrate body, mind, and spirit. The system of Integral Yoga was brought to the West from India by Sri Swami Satchidananda. This system emphasizes the practices of hatha yoga, pranayama, and meditation as the way to develop physical and mental stillness in order to unlock inner truth. Integral Yoga is practiced and taught at the Integral Yoga Institute, which was founded by Sri Swami Satchidananda and has branches throughout the United States and the rest of the world. Integral Yoga hatha classes are offered by individual teachers, by the Integral Yoga Institutes and Integral Yoga Teaching Centers, as well as at Integral Yoga headquarters at Satchidananda Ashram-Yogaville, which is located in Buckingham, near Charlottesville, Virginia.

The Origins of Integral Yoga

The founding and inspirational force behind Integral Yoga is Sri Swami Satchidananda. Born in South India, Sri Swami Satchidananda studied yoga under the guidance of several of the most renowned teachers of yoga in the 20th century, including Sri Ramana Maharashi, Sri Aurobindo, and, most especially, Sri Swami Sivananda. Sri Swami Sivananda of the city of Rishikesh in the Himalayas, who taught a synthesis of many different types of yoga, was

Sri Swami Satchidananda's spiritual master. Sri Swami Sivananda was one of the most influential teachers of yoga in the 20th century. He counted among his students Sri Swami Satchidananda, as well as Sri Swami Chidananda, Sri Swami Jyotirmayananda, and Sri Swami Vishnudevananda, who is responsible for the development of Sivananda Yoga (see Chapter 5).

Sri Swami Satchidananda traveled and taught extensively throughout Southeast Asia and Europe, and there are now yoga teachers and centers devoted to him throughout the world. He was invited to visit the West by an American devotee in 1966. A planned two-day visit turned into a five-month teaching tour. He quickly gained prominence as a teacher of yoga. Many Baby Boomers may remember him as the spiritual mentor of the 1969 Woodstock music festival. His 1970 guide to the practice of hatha yoga, *Integral Yoga Hatha*, introduced countless Westerners to yoga. It continues to remain a classic among texts on hatha yoga.

Integral Yoga is an integrative approach to yoga that is both systematic and practical. It was developed by Sri Swami Satchidananda, a student of Sri Swami Sivananda, whose teachings also contributed to the development of Sivananda Yoga. Born in South India, Sri Swami Satchidananda came to the United States in the 1960s. He gained popular recognition as the spiritual mentor of the 1969 Woodstock Music and Art Fair. Through its headquarters in Buckingham, Virginia, and branches and centers throughout the rest of the United States and the world, Integral Yoga offers classes and workshops that emphasize the accessibility and practicality of yoga. It uses hatha yoga to serve people seeking relief from stress and fatigue as a doorway to yoga practice. Formal classes are generally 75 to 90 minutes in length. Integral Yoga emphasizes ease and comfort in the performance of asanas. Pranayama and meditation receive equal weighting with asana practice within the Integral Yoga system.

Sri Swami Satchidananda founded the Integral Yoga Institute as the vehicle to teach his particular approach to yoga. Satchidananda Ashram-Yogaville, located in Buckingham, Virginia, is the international headquarters of Integral Yoga, and there are Integral Yoga branches and centers throughout the world. Integral Yoga remains one of the premier yoga organizations in the world today. It is one of the leading centers for the training of yoga teachers with more than 15 teacher training programs conducted at Yogaville each year. In addition, the New York, New Jersey, and San Francisco centers also conduct training. Teacher training programs in Gibraltar and Portugal conduct training for European teachers.

The Theory Underlying Integral Yoga

Integral Yoga represents a rich synthesis of the major principles of yoga. This style of yoga is characterized by its practical, simple, and systematic approach to the practice of yoga. Dean Ornish, M.D., who is famous for developing his healthy lifestyle program for reversing heart disease, studied Integral Yoga. It is this approach to yoga that forms one of the key components in his healthy lifestyle program.

The three foundational practices of Integral Yoga are asana practice, pranayama, and meditation. Practice of the physical asana postures purifies, aligns, and strengthens the body.

Pranayama, or the practice of breath control, is used to draw the mind and senses inward in order to progress up the higher rungs of the eight-limbed ladder of yoga. Meditation allows practitioners to connect to the divinity within.

The Integral Yoga approach to yoga emphasizes the accessibility and practicality of this ancient practice. It recognizes that many people come to yoga seeking relief from stress and fatigue. Integral Yoga uses hatha yoga as a doorway to yoga practice. The emphasis is on ease and comfort in performing the asanas. Pranayama and meditation receive equal weighting with asana practice within the Integral Yoga system.

In addition to these foundational practices, Integral Yoga teaches a variety of other practices and principles that are associated with a yoga lifestyle. These include relaxation techniques, vegetarian diet and cooking, as well as a yoga lifestyle training program.

Integral Yoga: The Style

Integral Yoga hatha is typically taught in a class setting. Classes are divided into levels of difficulty and include New Beginners, Beginners (Level I), Intermediate (Level II), and Advanced (Level III). Classes are generally open to anyone, with drop-ins encouraged.

Each Integral Yoga class follows a prescribed format. They are generally 75 to 90 minutes in length. The first 55 minutes are devoted to the practice of physical asanas, followed by a deep relaxation. Pranayama followed by meditation and a brief chanting session complete the class.

In addition to classes in asana practice, Integral Yoga Institutes and Teaching Centers offer a wide range of informative programs that range from individual lectures to ongoing courses, intense workshops, and residential retreats. Some sample topics include "HIV and Yoga," "Yoga and Psychotherapy," and classes in vegetarian cooking.

Background and Training of Practitioners

Training and certification in Integral Yoga is provided through the Integral Yoga Teacher Training Program. The Institute's Basic Hatha Yoga Teacher Training Program is offered at certain branch locations of the Integral Yoga Institute as an ongoing program that takes place over a number of months or as an intensive month-long residential training at its Buckingham, Virginia, headquarters. In addition to basic teacher training programs, programs in Intermediate Hatha Yoga Teacher Training, Advanced Hatha Yoga Teacher Training, Extra Gentle Yoga Teacher Training, and Yoga for the Special Child Teacher Training are offered annually at the Buckingham headquarters.

The Integral Yoga Basic Hatha Yoga Teacher Training Program is offered in several different formats. At Satchidananda Ashram-Yogaville it is available either as a month-long residential program or as a split session composed of two-week sessions in spring and fall. The Integral Yoga Institutes and Teaching Centers around the country also offer the program in one or both formats.

The curriculum of the Integral Yoga's Basic Hatha Yoga Teacher Training Program is designed to provide complete instruction in how to teach Integral Yoga Hatha Beginners I classes. Beginners I classes include hatha yoga postures, pranayama, meditation, and deep relaxation postures according to the teachings of Sri Swami Satchidananda. Attention is given to other aspects of yoga so that graduates have a full understanding of the complete scope of yoga. Subjects include anatomy and physiology, diet and nutrition, and the various branches of yoga. Participants learn how to organize and initiate classes, as well as deepen their own personal practice of yoga.

Integral Yoga has certified more than 2,000 teachers through this training program. Graduates of its program teach in every state, as well as in many foreign countries.

For further information on the Integral Yoga Teacher Training Program, contact:

Satchidananda Ashram—Yogaville
Teacher Certification Programs
Buckingham, VA 23921
Tel: (800) 858-9642

For Further Information

One of the best ways to find out more about Integral Yoga is to visit the Website maintained by Yogaville. This site contains information on Integral Yoga, the Integral Yoga programs, general information on yoga, links to Integral Yoga institutes and Integral Yoga teaching centers locations, and other recommended yoga resources on the Internet. The site also features a searchable database of certified Integral Yoga instructors both in the United States and worldwide. For further information on Integral Yoga, its branches, and programs, contact:

Satchidananda Ashram—Yogaville
Route 1, Box 1720
Buckingham, VA 23921
Tel: (434) 969-3121
Fax: (434) 969-1303
Website: *www.Yogaville.org*
E-mail: iyi@Yogaville.org

Integral Yoga Publications publishes a number of books on Integral Yoga, many by Sri Swami Satchidananda. In addition, Satchidananda Ashram-Yogaville operates a book distribution company that offers a wide variety of books and tapes on yoga and allied subjects by mail order. For further information, contact:

Integral Yoga Distribution
Satchidananda Ashram-Yogaville
Route 1, Box 1720
Buckingham, VA 23921
Website: *www.yogahealthbooks.com*
Tel: (800) 262-1008 or (434) 969-1049 (local calls)

Suggested Further Resources

Sri Swami Satchidananda has been a prolific teacher on the philosophy and practice of Integral Yoga. *Integral Yoga Magazine*, founded by Sri Swami Satchidananda in 1970, is the official journal of Integral Yoga and Sri Swami Satchidananda's teachings. Published quarterly, subscriptions are available by going online to *www.Yogaville.org* or requesting a subscription form by calling Yogaville. Sri Swami Satchidananda's teachings on the philosophy and practice of Integral Yoga have been compiled into a large number of books. A complete listing of his titles in print can be obtained by contacting Integral Yoga Distribution. The following list of books is provided to help you get started in learning more about the fundamentals of Integral Yoga:

Sri Swami Satchidananda, *Integral Yoga Hatha* (Integral Yoga Publications, 1995). This clear and comprehensive, illustrated yoga manual remains a classic introduction to hatha yoga.

————, *The Yoga Sutras of Patanjali: Translation and Commentary on the Raja Yoga Sutras* (Integral Yoga Publications, 1978). In this commentary on and translation of the classic treatise on yoga, Sri Swami Satchidananda offers practical advice based on his experience and the practice of Integral Yoga.

The following is an inspiring biography of Sri Swami Satchidananda:

Sita Bordow, *Swami Satchidananda: Apostle of Peace* (Integral Yoga Publications, 1986). This richly illustrated biography chronicles Sri Swami Satchidananda's life, from his beginnings in South India to meetings with global leaders.

The following tapes are recommended for those individuals who would like to begin the practice of Integral Yoga:

Sri Swami Satchidananda, *Integral Hatha Yoga* (Integral Yoga Publications). In this 80-minute videotape, Sri Swami Satchidananda guides the viewer through a session of Integral Yoga, including 45 minutes of yoga postures and a guided deep relaxation.

Integral Yoga Hatha Tapes (Integral Yoga Publishers). An entire series of audiotapes are available to help guide you through many of the levels of practice of Integral Yoga. This selection includes a 30-minute tape for those with limited time and a tape on Extra Gentle Integral Yoga, among many other offerings available.

Swami Ramananda on yoga for men:

"While I think that yoga is certainly helpful for everyone, yoga is particularly beneficial for men because of the way it can counteract some unhealthy male tendencies and reeducate us as men. In so many ways, our educational system has conditioned us to value ourselves based on what we produce. Most men are identified with their jobs, valuing themselves according to what they earn, by their title, status, or possessions. Society trains us to value our image even over how we feel. As a result, men experience a deeply rooted but unspoken stress that they should be more or better than who they are. Yoga counteracts this conditioning because the goal of yoga is to be in touch with ourselves as spiritual beings, to appreciate deeper

(Continued)

aspects of our human experience such as being at peace, having loving relationships, and simply enjoying life. Yoga can teach us that these experiences ultimately are not dependent on things outside of ourselves such as having things go just right or winning the admiration of others.

"Many men approach yoga through the physical practices of hatha yoga. If a hatha class is taught in a traditional way, we perform the postures free of any need to accomplish something or live up to an image. We practice by learning to listen and accept the capacity of the body as it is. So rather than imposing on the body how it should be, hatha practice guides us to move according to our ability at each moment and to respond to what we encounter in ourselves with respect and compassion. This is a powerful antidote to the pressure of maintaining an image that tends to drive men's lives.

"In hatha yoga, we grow our practice by becoming truly aware of where we are in the present moment. In each asana, we learn to progress by coming mindfully in touch with our limits and holding each pose carefully without causing strain. Similarly, to grow out of bad habits, we need to look deeply at what forces are compelling us and know clearly where we are, so that we can see what new step to take and take it with awareness and care. The 'just do it' approach that our culture impresses upon men amounts to forcing ourselves to change and rarely produces lasting results.

"Our yoga practice also teaches us to achieve a balance of effort and ease—to act with a mind that is both energized and calm, focused yet free of anxiousness. This mental state is ideal for doing just about anything we undertake and is especially conducive to clarity and creativity.

"Integral Yoga hatha is a unique style that is grounded in the ultimate goal of realizing one's full potential. It may be less physically challenging than some other styles of yoga, but it is perhaps more psychologically challenging for men, because it asks of them to move free of concern for how they look, and instead to focus on what they feel. Thus, the goal of Integral Yoga hatha is to create ease in the body and peace in the mind versus achieving some ideal physical condition.

"Longer term, our yoga practice helps us remove the obstacles to experiencing our natural state of vitality and steadiness on the physical and mental levels. The ultimate benefits come when the body and the mind are able to be still enough to begin to experience the spiritual level of our being, giving rise to innate feelings of peace, fulfillment, and happiness that are not dependent on anything outside of us. As we become established in the awareness of our true nature, life becomes joyful and we are capable of giving and serving others in meaningful ways."

—Swami Ramananda, President of the Integral Yoga Institute of New York

Chapter 4

IYENGAR YOGA

Iyengar's Dynamic Precision

When your body, mind, and soul are healthy and harmonious, you will bring health and harmony to those around you and health and harmony to the world—not by withdrawing from the world but by being a healthy living organ of the body of humanity.[1]

—B.K.S. Iyengar

What Is Iyengar Yoga?

Iyengar Yoga is an approach to yoga developed by Bellur Kirshnamachar Sundararaja Iyengar, known more commonly as B.K.S. Iyengar (1918–). It aims to integrate body, mind, and soul. Iyengar Yoga is known for the dynamic precision that its practitioners exemplify in their execution of the physical asanas. It is a complete system of yoga that aims to liberate the soul by integrating the mind and the body through the practice of asanas. In Iyengar Yoga, asana practice becomes meditation in motion, and yoga itself becomes "the perfect art in action."[2]

The Origins of Iyengar Yoga

While Iyengar Yoga is based on the time-honored traditions of yoga practice, the specific way in which it approaches the practice and teaching of yoga is the result of Iyengar's lifetime of practice, observation, and teaching of yoga.

Iyengar was born in 1918 in South India. As a boy, he experienced a number of health complaints, which eventually sent him (in 1934) to seek instruction in yoga. His teacher was Krishnamacharya, Iyengar's brother-in-law and one of the most celebrated teachers of yoga in India at the time. Krishnamacharya, who was head of the Yoga Institute at the Royal Palace of Mysore, was also teacher to several other noted yoga masters of this century, including his own son, T.K.V. Desikachar, who has been very influential in the West through the work of his American student, Gary Kraftsow, who teaches Viniyoga (page 107); and K. Pattabhi Jois, who developed Ashtanga Yoga (page 67), popularized as Power Yoga.

Iyengar began to teach yoga in 1936. Interestingly enough, Iyengar reports that

> Iyengar Yoga was developed by B.K.S. Iyengar (1918–), one of the most influential teachers of yoga in the world. Iyengar Yoga is renowned for its emphasis on precision and artistry in the execution of physical postures. Iyengar paid particular attention to the relation of yoga to anatomy, physiology, and pathology. As a result, his style of yoga incorporates an extensive system of props, such as cloth straps, wooden or foam blocks, blankets, and bolsters, to help practitioners achieve better and more comfortable balance and alignment when performing asanas. During an Iyengar Yoga class, the teacher pays great attention to instructing students as specifically as possible in how to perform each posture.

in the 1930s, it was difficult to find students of yoga, even in India.[3] Fortunately for ensuing generations, Iyengar did eventually find students, and has continued to refine his approach to yoga over the decades. Iyengar has perfected the practice of more than 200 asanas and breathing techniques. In 1974, Iyengar visited the United States for the first time and introduced the West to his particular style of yoga. Over the course of his lifetime, millions of students have studied his Iyengar Yoga. He currently lives in Pune, India, where he presides over his own institute, the Ramamani Iyengar Memorial Institute (RIMYI), which he established in 1975 in loving memory of his deceased wife. His daughter, Geeta, and son, Prashant, who collaborate as teachers and researchers into the history and philosophy of yoga, have joined him in his work.

Iyengar Yoga is celebrated for the precision that it brings to the practice of yoga. Among the many gifts that Iyengar has offered to yoga is the unceasing intellectual clarity that he has brought to bear upon the practice of yoga. Iyengar himself suffered from many illnesses as a child, including malaria, typhoid, and tuberculosis.[4] Owing to his own health concerns as well as those of his students over the years, he has paid particular care to the relation of yoga to anatomy, physiology, and pathology. He has had the opportunity to work with people who have many and various physical ailments, and thus has designed a style of yoga that can address many health concerns. He considers yoga a therapy as well as a philosophy. His work has been much praised by the medical establishment.

Because he has had so much experience in dealing with people with physical limitations (which includes nearly everyone), Iyengar developed a unique way of providing assistance to practitioners of yoga in the form of yoga props, or accessories. For instance, wood or foam blocks can be placed on the floor to provide balance and support for standing postures that require the practitioner to place a hand on the floor. A belt looped around the feet and held in the hands can ease strain in performing a seated forward bend. Placing a bolster or blanket under the buttocks can help you to feel more comfortable while sitting in a cross-legged sitting position. The teachers of many styles of yoga now use such props. However, it was Iyengar, with his emphasis on the precise anatomical alignment of the body while performing yoga, who popularized these powerful aids.

The Theory Underlying Iyengar Yoga

A man's original state is one of wholeness and harmony of body, mind, and spirit. However, time and the stresses of life tend to make men's lives scattered and fragmented. Iyengar Yoga aims to help practitioners achieve the ultimate goal of yoga: unification of body, mind, and spirit.

Yoga is an immense system. It is an art, a science, a philosophy, a discipline, and a therapy. Iyengar likens yoga to a tree, which he calls the tree of yoga. He likens each of the eight steps of yoga (see Chapter 1) to a part of a tree. Yamas ("abstentions") are the roots of the tree. Niyamas ("restraints") are the trunk. The various asanas ("postures") form the many branches of the tree. Pranayama ("regulation of the breath") practices are the leaves, which interface between the external and internal worlds. Pratyahara ("withdrawal of the senses") forms the bark of the tree. Dharana ("concentration") is the life sap of the tree. Dhyana ("meditation") is the flower of the tree. Samadhi ("ecstasy") is the final offering of the tree—its fruit.[5]

The asanas, or physical postures, of the tree of yoga are considered vitally important because they are meant to bring the body to its greatest state of well-being. They prepare the body to receive the inflow of vital life force that pranayama practices promote. The asanas also allow the mind to unite in consciousness with the body so that self-realization can take place. When mindfully performed, asana practice is meditation, which leads to self-realization.

Iyengar Yoga: The Style

Iyengar Yoga is most frequently taught in a class setting, although, as in most styles of yoga, private instruction with a teacher is generally widely available. Classes typically last from 60 to 90 minutes. They are typically ranked by level of difficulty and the background of the students.

During an Iyengar Yoga class, the teacher pays great attention to instructing students as specifically as possible in how to perform each asana. This may entail the instructor's demonstrating the proper way to execute the asana first, then having the students follow. Once the students have performed the asana a first time, the instructor might then demonstrate the pose again, pointing out a deeper subtlety and specificity of the pose. Students then repeat the asana. This process may continue for several rounds until the students become even more precise in their repetition of the asana. Often, the teacher will focus on just one aspect of an asana in order to bring full awareness to its execution. For instance, a teacher may focus on just one position in the Sun Salutation series, such as Downward-Facing Dog Pose, in order to emphasize the correct form in holding the position. (For more information on this yoga sequence of movements, see "A Complete Yoga Practice Session for Men.")

In order to assist students further in their asana practice, teachers of Iyengar Yoga also often incorporate rich visual imagery into their speech as they talk students through the execution of a posture. This imagery has the effect of taking the student deeper into the pose, as well as allowing the student's mind to become engaged in the pose, thus promoting yoga's goal of uniting body and mind.

Classes in Iyengar Yoga often incorporate the props and accessories discussed earlier in this chapter. For instance, while performing Triangle Pose (see Fig. YPS.4b, page 123), a teacher might encourage a student to use a wood or sturdy foam block for support. In the Triangle Pose, a student stands with his legs several feet apart while lifting the torso to one side as one hand is raised toward the ceiling and the other is placed on the floor. For many students, it is difficult to lower the hand onto the floor without losing the form of the pose. Placing a prop on the floor provides added height that allows the student to perform the pose without compromising the integrity of his form.

Iyengar Yoga is often considered a dynamic form of yoga. In fact, movements can range from very gentle to rather active. In general, beginning students use slower, gentler movements, and hold postures for a shorter period of time. As they progress in their practice of Iyengar Yoga, postures become more complex and are held for longer periods of time. The quality of dynamism is most appropriately applied to the dynamic interplay between mind and body while performing asana practice. It is this connection of mind and body that makes Iyengar Yoga meditation in motion, and enables the practitioner to be at one in body, mind, and spirit.

Iyengar Yoga is particularly beneficial for those individuals who are interested in detailed, precise instruction in performance of the asanas. These instructions are geared to take the student from beginning to advanced postures in a systematic, step-by-step fashion.

Iyengar Yoga can be especially helpful for those individuals who are suffering from a particular health problem and wish to help resolve it through the practice of yoga. Iyengar views yoga as therapy. He studied the physiological effects that yoga has on the body and applied the practice of yoga to the treatment of a host of medical conditions, such as liver and stomach problems, psoriasis, muscular complaints, and eye and hearing problems. These are just a few of the many conditions for which Iyengar Yoga has been used.

Iyengar is clear in encouraging students to begin their practice of yoga gradually and within the limits of their abilities. Because Iyengar has specialized in developing methods for helping people modify postures in accordance with their physical limitations, Iyengar Yoga may be especially well suited to men with particular disabilities. Older men may also benefit from Iyengar Yoga's extensive use of props, whose support can help them execute postures that might otherwise be difficult or impossible.

Background and Training of Teachers

The B.K.S. Iyengar Yoga National Association of the United States, Inc. (IYNAUS), oversees training of teachers in Iyengar Yoga. This training is designed to ensure that Iyengar Yoga teachers have a mature knowledge and regular practice of this discipline. An Iyengar Yoga teacher instructs yoga in the method set forth by B.K.S. Iyengar without mixing in other styles of yoga or other disciplines; receives continuing instruction from the RIMYI in

Pune, India, or from intermediate or advanced Iyengar teachers; acknowledges the governing influence of the teaching of B.K.S. Iyengar on his or her practice and teaching of yoga; and maintains a regular personal practice of Iyengar Yoga. Training as a teacher of Iyengar Yoga generally takes at least two years to complete, and is one of the most rigorous in the field of yoga.

For Further Information

The B.K.S. Iyengar National Association of the United States Inc. (IYNAUS) is the central clearinghouse for information on Iyengar Yoga teachers in the United States. At its Website, you'll find information on Iyengar Yoga, including biographical information regarding Iyengar, guidelines for teacher certification, a searchable database of Iyengar Yoga teachers worldwide, and links to regional and international Iyengar Yoga associations. IYNAUS is staffed by volunteers, with regional associations in different parts of the country. The best way to obtain further information is to call its toll-free telephone number or visit its Website:

B.K.S. Iyengar National Association of the United States Inc.

Tel: (800) 889-9642 (YOGA)

Website: *www.iynaus.org*

The B.K.S. Iyengar Institute in Pune, India, maintains an official Website with valuable information on Iyengar Yoga:

B.K.S. Iyengar Institute

Website: *www.bksiyengar.com*

E-mail: mehtat@vsnl.com

Suggested Further Resources

B.K.S. Iyengar has written prolifically on the subject of yoga. The following are among his principal books:

B.K.S. Iyengar, *Light on Yoga, Revised Edition* (Schocken Books, 1977). This is Iyengar's classic text on yoga and his unique approach to it, complete with more than 600 black-and-white photographs of him demonstrating the physical postures.

————, *Light on Pranayama: The Yogic Art of Breathing* (Crossroad, 1997). This is Iyengar's classic text on the yogic science of breathing, prefaced by an overview of yoga philosophy.

————, *The Tree of Yoga* (Shambhala, 1988). Based on Iyengar's lectures and discussions with his students, this book presents Iyengar's insights into a variety of subjects, including the metaphysical and historical roots of yoga, yoga's role today, and yoga's relationship to health, family, and other matters.

————, *Yoga: The Path to Holistic Health* (Dorling Kindersley, 2001). This is Iyengar's updated and complete guide to his system of yoga, lavishly illustrated and with complete sample yoga programs to suit virtually any man's needs.

In addition to Iyengar's own books, the following book is recommended:

Mira Silva and Mehta Shyam, *Yoga: The Iyengar Way* (Alfred A. Knopf, 1990). This book, written by a family team that has studied and taught Iyengar Yoga for more than 30 years, is a beautifully illustrated introduction to Iyengar Yoga, with clear and precise instructions on how to perform more than 100 asanas. This book contains detailed information on which postures are beneficial for specific health concerns.

B.K.S. Iyengar on yoga and your health:

"Disease is an offensive force; inner energy is a defensive force. As we grow, the defensive strength gets less and the offensive strength increases. That is how diseases enter into our system. A body which carries out yogic practice is like a fort which keeps up its defensive strength so that the offensive strength in the form of diseases will not enter into it through the skin. Which do you prefer? Yoga helps to maintain the defensive strength at an optimum level, and that is what is known as health."[6]

—B.K.S. Iyengar, Yoga Master and Teacher of his own
signature approach to yoga

Chapter 5

SIVANANDA YOGA

Swami Vishnu-devananda's Classical Five-Point System

Serve. Love. Give. Purify. Meditate. Realize.[1]

—Swami Sivananda

What Is Sivananda Yoga?

Sivananda Yoga is a classical system of yoga developed by Sri Swami Vishnu-devananda (1927–1993). It is based on a five-point system that can help men develop physical, mental, and spiritual health by promoting proper exercise, breathing, relaxation, diet, and positive thinking (*vedanta*) and meditation to achieve physical, mental, and spiritual well-being.

The Origins of Sivananda Yoga

Sivananda Yoga represents Swami Vishnu-devananda's practical implementation of raja yoga and vedanta philosophy. Swami Vishnu-devananda was a student of Swami Sivananda (1887–1963), for whom this approach to yoga is named and upon whose teachings it is based. Born in Pattamadai, Tamil Nadu, South India, Swami Sivananda served many years as a medical doctor before devoting himself exclusively to the practice and teaching of yoga. His approach to yoga represents a synthesis of classic yoga teachings, integrating the principles of the four main yoga traditions of India: bhakti yoga, jnana yoga, karma yoga, and raja yoga (see Chapter 1). Author of more than 300 books, Swami Sivananda founded the Divine Life Society and established the Sivananda Ashram in Rishikesh, North India.

Swami Vishnu-devananda, who was one of Swami Sivananda's most fervent and adept students, was born in Kerala, South India. Swami Sivananda sent this young protégé to North America in 1957 with a 10 rupee note and the simple encouragement: "People are waiting."[2] Swami Vishnu-devananda designed a practical five-point system in order to make the teachings of yoga and vedanta more accessible in the West. He implemented this system through his teaching, writing, and founding of the International Sivananda Yoga Vedanta Centres in Montreal, Canada, in 1959. His seminal text, *The Complete Illustrated Book of Yoga*, which was published in 1960 and is still extensively read today, brought these teachings to widespread attention. His sensible and simple-to-follow approach to yoga gained many adherents and made what had seemed an esoteric Eastern approach accessible.

The Theory Underlying Sivananda Yoga

The ultimate goal of Sivananda Yoga is to enable us to maintain control over the mind. According to the adherents of this approach to yoga, only when the mind is stable can we be calm, centered, and at peace. In common with other approaches to yoga, the teachings of Sivananda Yoga maintain that much of our discontent and illness stems from imbalance and lack of control. We become attached to external objects and lose our true sense of self and focus. The ultimate goal of Sivananda Yoga is to develop stillness of mind so that we can be at peace under any circumstances.

This goal is not so easy to achieve, though. The mind is very hard to control. It has a tendency to be scattered by uncontrollable thoughts and emotions. Sivananda Yoga aims to help develop control of the mind through a complete five-point system comprised of the following disciplines:

1. Proper exercise (*asanas*, or yoga postures). Proper exercise is introduced in hatha yoga courses. These courses teach a series of yoga postures that help stretch and strengthen the body, improve circulation, and promote proper functioning of the internal organs and glands. In addition, they help develop control over the body and nervous system in preparation for proper relaxation and meditation.

2. Proper breathing (*pranayama*). In Sanskrit, the breath is called *prana* and it refers not only to

Sivananda Yoga is based on the teachings of the revered Indian saint, Sri Swami Sivananda (1887–1963). It is characterized by a simple and well-balanced synthesis of the four main traditions of yoga—bhakti yoga, jnana yoga, karma yoga, and raja yoga. It is based upon a five-point system that can help men develop physical, mental and spiritual health by promoting proper exercise, proper breathing, proper relaxation, proper diet, and positive thinking and meditation. This system was designed by Swami Vishnu-devananda (1927–1993), a student of Swami Sivananda, to make the classical teachings of yoga more accessible to the Western audience. Swami Vishnu-devananda helped spread these teachings by founding the International Sivananda Yoga Vedanta Centres in 1959. Sivananda Yoga is one of the most widely studied and practiced styles of yoga in the world today. With close to 80 centers worldwide, the International Yoga Vedanta Centers have trained more than 15,000 teachers of yoga.

breath, but also to vital life energy. *Pranayama*, or the science of breath, teaches specific breathing exercises that help to stabilize the body and mind. In addition, it recharges and balances the nervous system and the flow of life energy through subtle pathways in the body.

3. Proper relaxation (*savasana*). Proper relaxation helps us to absorb the many benefits that are derived from yoga practice. It also helps to release tension and toxins from the body. Often, in our own lives, we deplete our energy during our so-called leisure time in frenetic pursuit of what we call, perhaps mistakenly, "relaxation" activities—such as staying up late reveling or club-crawling. Sivananda Yoga teaches proper relaxation techniques, which conserve energy and quiet the body, mind, and spirit.

4. Proper diet (vegetarian). Proper diet is essential to the optimum functioning of both body and mind. Sivananda Yoga advocates maintaining a simple, vegetarian diet of mainly organically grown food that eschews spices, intoxicating beverages, caffeine, and heavy food—all of which slow the body down. Such a diet can be tastefully prepared and can satisfy all of our needs.

5. Positive thinking (*vedanta*) and meditation. *Vedanta* literally means the "end of the *Vedas*" and refers to the metaphysical wisdom contained in the *Upanishads*, which are the final parts of the *Vedas*.[3] Meditation enables us to still the mind so we are able to contact our Timeless Self and find true happiness. Such happiness is not dependent on the vagaries of the external world.

Sivananda Yoga: The Style

Sivananda Yoga is one of the most widely practiced approaches to yoga. It is taught at nearly 80 Sivananda locations (ashrams, yoga centers, and affiliated centers) throughout the United States and the rest of the world. More than 15,000 teachers of yoga throughout the world have been trained in this approach to yoga.

Typically, Sivananda Yoga is taught in several courses that progress from beginner to intermediate and advanced. Beginners Yoga, Part I, is a five-session class that focuses on proper exercise (basic yoga postures), proper breathing, and proper relaxation. Each class is 60 minutes in length. Instruction is continued in Beginners Yoga, Part 2, which teaches the rest of the basic yoga postures and exercises, and introduces the principles of proper diet, positive thinking, and meditation. This course is also a five-class series, with each class lasting 90 minutes. Additional classes are offered in intermediate and advanced yoga postures, as well as in meditation.

Once students have completed the two beginners' courses, they are free to attend open classes, which are typical of a Sivananda Yoga class. These classes last for 90 minutes and follow a prescribed protocol. They begin with approximately 20 minutes of two basic breathing exercises. Breathing exercises are followed by more than an hour of physical exercises, which are comprised of 12 basic yoga postures. Each class concludes with a long, deep relaxation.

In addition to instruction in classic Sivananda Yoga, a variety of classes are frequently available that are tailored to specific needs. For instance, Gentle Yoga, performed in chairs, can be especially helpful for seniors and the physically impaired. A Headstand Workshop can help you to develop stability in performing headstands while overcoming fear. Yoga for Kids presents yoga to children 7 to 13 years of age. In addition, a wide range of classes and workshops are offered in vegetarian cooking, yogic cleansing practices, yogic breathing, and other topics related to health and well-being.

Background and Training of Teachers

Upon successful completion of the first-level course of teacher training and examination, teachers of Sivananda Yoga receive a diploma from the Sivananda Yoga Vedanta Centers and Ashrams, which is a copy of the original diploma Swami Sivananda used to issue to his disciples at the Yoga Vedanta Forest Academy of Rishikesh, India. This first level of training is comprised of an intensive, four-week residential program in the theory and practice of all aspects of yoga. The program is offered throughout the year at a variety of retreat centers (ashrams) located at numerous sites in the United States, Canada, the Caribbean, Europe, India, and throughout the rest of the world.

The Sivananda Yoga teacher training program was developed by Swami Vishnu-devananda. The first level includes instruction in such various yoga practices as yoga postures, breathing exercises, cleansing techniques, proper diet, meditation, mantra, yoga philosophy, and anatomy and physiology. In addition, an advanced yoga teacher training course is offered once a year.

You should be able to find a teacher of Sivananda Yoga near you: Since 1968, when Swami Vishnu-devananda created the first yoga teacher training course ever taught in the West, more than 15,000 teachers of yoga have been trained worldwide in accordance with the teachings of Swami Sivananda.

For Further Information

With more than 345 pages, the Sivananda Yoga Website (*www.sivananda.org*) is one of the most extensive sources of yoga information available on the Internet. By visiting the site, you can find comprehensive information regarding the teachings of yoga; the various activities of the Sivananda Yoga centers throughout the United States and the rest of the world; Sivananda Yoga teacher training courses; recommended books and other supplemental materials; and an online yoga boutique. The site contains innovative enhancements, such as interactive, animated instruction in the chakras for those who are interested in the subtle energy anatomy of yoga (see Chapter 7) and downloadable files of yoga screensavers that may appeal to the techie in you. Information is available on the Website in English, French, German, and Spanish.

If you do not have access to the Web, the Sivananda Yoga Vedanta Center in New York City acts as a clearinghouse for information on Sivananda Yoga in the United States:

The Sivananda Yoga Vedanta Center
243 West 24th Street
New York, NY 10011
Tel: (212) 255-4560

Fax: (212) 2727-7392

E-mail: NewYork@Sivananda.org

The worldwide headquarters of Sivananda Yoga Vedanta Center is located in Val-Morin, Quebec, Canada, one hour's drive north of Montreal.

International Sivananda Yoga Centres

673 Eighth Avenue

Val Morin, Quebec, JOT 2RO

Canada

Tel: (819) 322-3226 (in Canada) or (800) 263-YOGA (toll-free)

Fax: (819) 322-5876

E-mail: HQ@sivananda.org

Additional Sivananda Yoga Vedanta Centers and Ashrams are located throughout North America, including the United States, Canada, and the Bahamas, as well as in Argentina, Australia, Austria, France, Germany, India, Israel, Spain, Switzerland, Uruguay, and the United Kingdom.

Suggested Further Resources

The following are recommended books and videos on Sivananda Yoga:

Sivananda Yoga Center, *The Sivananda Companion to Yoga* (Simon and Schuster, 1983). An easy-to-read, illustrated introduction to the five-point system of Sivananda Yoga.

————, *Yoga Mind & Body* (DK Publishing, Inc., 1996). A beautifully photographed, full-color, over-sized book summarizing the Sivananda Yoga Vedanta philosophy. Includes detailed descriptions of the physical exercise poses, and delicious, healthy vegetarian recipes. This book is an excellent introduction to the general principles of yoga.

Swami Vishnu-devananda, *The Complete Illustrated Book of Yoga* (Crown, 1960). This is the classic introduction to Sivananda Yoga, including the history and theory of yoga practices, a practical guide to yoga postures and practices, and sample programs for people of various ages and physical constitutions. It is profusely illustrated with black-and-white photographs of yoga exercises.

The Sivananda Yoga Video: For the do-it-yourselfer, a complete video guide to the techniques and practice of Sivananda Yoga lushly photographed at the Sivananda Yoga retreat on Paradise Island in the Bahamas. Features expert demonstration. It runs for 59 minutes.

In addition, audiotapes, training manuals, magazines, and brochures are available by contacting the Sivananda Yoga Vedanta Centres.

Swami Sadasivananda on yoga for men:

"We are living in the age in which we witness a tremendous amount of transformation taking place on all levels and in all areas of our lives. As result of it, we are undergoing incredible changes both without and within us which in turn creates stress for our body and mind. Yoga is one of the most effective means to combat the side-effects of fast living and balance the transformation which it carries. In order to live in harmony with the world and himself, every man should do his best to come in touch and reconnect with his body, mind, and the deeper, spiritual aspect of his being. The synthesis of proper exercise, proper breathing, proper relaxation, proper diet, and positive thinking and meditation applied in daily life is a *sine qua non* for right, harmonious, and joyous living. Men who dedicate some amount of time in the application of these ancient yogic disciplines will certainly regain their health, will have the abundance of energy, and live happily. They will regain their confidence, charisma, and ability to relate to the world in a spontaneous and compassionate way and live peacefully."

—Swami Sadasivananda, Director of the Sivananda Yoga Vedanta Center
in New York City

Chapter 6

ASHTANGA YOGA

Power Yoga

Eliminating impurity through continued practice of the eight limbs of yoga brings discernment and clear perception. The eight limbs of yoga are: respect toward others, self-restraint, posture, breath control, detaching at will from the senses, concentration, meditation, and contemplation.[1]

—Patanjali (*Yoga Sutras*, II, 28-29)

What Is Ashtanga Yoga?

Ashtanga Yoga (sometimes alternatively spelled "Astanga" Yoga) is a precise and systematic approach to yoga that emphasizes physical strength and endurance in executing a flowing series of prescribed yoga postures. Various bodily locks and seals are applied in conjunction with a special kind of yogic breathing and gazing with the eyes in a prescribed way at certain fixed points of vision. The combined effect of all these practices results in the generation of heat and energy in a uniquely invigorating and flowing approach to yoga. *Ashtanga* literally means "eight limbs" in Sanskrit. This style of yoga is named for the eight-limbed path of yoga outlined by Patanjali in his *Yoga Sutras* (see page 35). Because this style of yoga is characterized by an especially vigorous approach to practicing the asanas of yoga, it is sometimes popularly referred to as "Power Yoga."

The Origins of Ashtanga Yoga

The origins of Ashtanga Yoga are the stuff of which myths and legends are made. This particular system of yoga is believed to have originated thousands of years ago, yet its

Ashtanga Yoga (sometimes alternatively spelled "Astanga" Yoga) is a precise and systematic approach to yoga that emphasizes physical strength and endurance in executing a flowing series of prescribed yoga postures. Various bodily locks and seals are applied in conjunction with a special kind of yogic breathing. The combined effect of all these practices results in the generation of heat and energy in a uniquely invigorating and flowing approach to yoga. *Ashtanga* literally means "eight limbs" in Sanskrit. This style of yoga is named for the eight-limbed path of yoga outlined by Patanjali in his seminal text on yoga, *Yoga Sutras.* Because this style of yoga is characterized by an especially vigorous approach to practicing the asanas of yoga, it is sometimes referred to as "Power Yoga."

modern-day rediscovery occurred only about 75 years ago. The individuals who are most responsible for having brought it into contemporary usage are East Indian yoga masters Sri Tirumlai Krishnamacharya (1888–1989) and Sri Krishna Pattabhi Jois (1915–). Krishnamacharya was one of the foremost yoga teachers of the 20th century. Founder and director of the Yoga School of Mysore, India, established in the Portrait Gallery in the Palace of the Maharaja of Mysore, his students included B.K.S. Iyengar (see Chapter 4), as well as his own son, T.K.V. Desikachar. Jois was one of the most devoted students of Krishnamacharya, with whom he studied privately for many years, as well as at the Mysore yoga school.

According to a frequently recounted story, Krishnamacharya is said to have come across an ancient text describing a series of yoga postures while on a visit to the National Library in Calcutta, India.[2] This text, *Yoga Korunta* by the sage Vamana Rishi, was particularly noteworthy because it described not only the asanas, or physical postures of yoga, but also the exact order and manner in which they were to be executed. The practices described in this text are believed to date back several thousand years. While descriptions of individual postures had been handed down within the yoga tradition, no text had ever been discovered that described an entire yoga practice sequence. No trace of the *Yoga Korunta* exists today, and Krishnamacharya is believed to have been the only individual in recent history to have direct knowledge of it.

This popular story is felt by many to be apocryphal. According to Jois, not only the *Yoga Korunta,* but also the *Hatha Yoga Pradipika,* the *Yoga Sutras,* and the *Bhagavad Gita* influenced the approach to yoga that Krishnamacharya taught Jois.[3] Jois, in turn, refined this system into a flowing practice sequence. Jois named his system Ashtanga Yoga because to him it represented the most complete embodiment of the eight-limbed (*ashtanga*) path of raja yoga.

Ashtanga Yoga was brought to the United States in the 1970s by a trio of young American seekers who had set off to India in search for the authentic practice of yoga.[4] When they saw Jois's son demonstrating his father's flowing Ashtanga Yoga sequences one day, they felt they had found what they were looking for. In 1972, the initial pioneers included Norman Allen and David Williams, who would eventually be joined by Nancy Gilgoff. Over the course of several years they studied Ashtanga Yoga directly with Jois, then returned to the West to teach it. They soon invited Jois to come and teach Ashtanga Yoga in the United States. Since that time, many in the West have embraced

Ashtanga Yoga and made the pilgrimage to Mysore, India, to experience and learn Ashtanga Yoga firsthand with Jois.

One of the most famous teachers of Ashtanga Yoga is Beryl Bender Birch. A teacher of yoga for many years, she studied with both Allen and Jois to perfect the practice of Ashtanga Yoga. As director of wellness for the New York Road Runner's Club, she shared this style of yoga with thousands of athletes around the world. Her best-selling book, *Power Yoga: The Total Strength and Flexibility Workout*, was the first book in English to detail the entire practice of Ashtanga Yoga. Through this book, Beryl Bender Birch helped introduce Ashtanga Yoga to people around the world. Ashtanga Yoga appeals to many men because of its power, grace, and ability to promote health, harmony, and balance. Many individuals around the globe now practice it.

The Theory Underlying Ashtanga Yoga

Despite the possible apocryphal nature of its origins, many practitioners of Ashtanga Yoga believe that Jois's approach represents the most complete and original system of yoga known. If it is indeed authentic, the manuscript of the *Yoga Korunta* is believed to be at least 1,500 years old, and the practices it describes are believed to be perhaps 5,000 years old. Some people even believe that Ashtanga Yoga embodies the original classical practice of yoga as referenced by Patanjali in his famous *Yoga Sutras*.

Ashtanga Yoga derives its name from the fact that practitioners believe it embodies all eight limbs of raja yoga, or the "royal" path to liberation. These limbs, which are presented in detail in Chapter 1, address a full spectrum of yoga principles, including right conduct, right action, physical movement, breathing, and the more abstract realms of sense withdrawal, contemplation, meditation, and ecstatic union with the absolute.

In addition to emphasizing learning and repeating a prescribed series of flowing asana postures, Ashtanga Yoga also incorporates a special breathing technique, bodily locks, and a special gazing technique. The practice of Ashtanga Yoga requires the exercising of moral observances, such as discipline and commitment. It can help lead men to a state of single-pointed concentration that is conducive to meditation. A man can experience the positive benefits of Ashtanga Yoga not only during physical execution of the series of postures, but also in his life in general. Thus, Ashtanga Yoga can be a gateway to living the yoga lifestyle.

Ashtanga Yoga differs from the other major styles of hatha yoga in a number of important respects. First, it incorporates a type of flowing movement known as *vinyasa* ("uninterrupted flow" or "arrangement" in Sanskrit). Each posture flows without interruption into the succeeding posture in a practice that is seamless and totally connected by the breath. This differs markedly from some other styles of yoga in which practitioners perform one asana, stop to rest, and then begin another. In addition, Ashtanga Yoga incorporates a special kind of breathing technique known as *ujjayi* ("victorious") breath. Ujjayi breath requires practitioners to constrict the passageways of the throat, resulting in a type of breathing that produces a hissing sound, even with the mouth closed. This breath helps to focus the mind as well as stoke heat in the body. Ashtanga Yoga also uses what are known as *bandhas* ("locks" in Sanskrit). Practitioners tighten certain internal muscles while performing Ashtanga Yoga—*mula bandha* ("root lock") draws up on the muscles of the pelvic floor and *uddiyana bandha* helps lock the area of the abdomen. Applying these yogic locks helps to seal in energy, focus awareness, and generate and retain heat and energy in the internal organs of the body. Fixing the gaze on certain prescribed points (*dristhi* or *drishti* in Sanskrit) helps to stabilize, purify, and concentrate the mind with single-pointed awareness. Ashtanga Yoga also requires strength to perform because various muscle groups are alternately and systematically contracted. Finally, to combine all of these features mindfully into one seamless flow requires a great deal of concentration. While other approaches to yoga may incorporate some of these techniques and principles, Ashtanga Yoga uses all of them in an integrated and dynamic approach to the practice of yoga.

The end result of the combination of practices that are used in Ashtanga Yoga is the generation of heat in the body and, in particular, the area of the abdomen. This heat has profound benefits, which range from the physical to the emotional, mental, and spiritual. The heat generated during the practice of Ashtanga Yoga helps to release tightness in muscles, ligaments, joints, and other parts of a man's body, as well as in the internal organs. The heat actually allows the tissues in the body to soften so that previously constricted areas can remold themselves into more appropriate alignment. The release of areas of physical holding can be accompanied by the letting go of tight, restricted, or outmoded ways of feeling and thinking as well.

In addition to its effects on the soft tissue of the body, the generation of heat can also play an important role in spiritual development. Yogis have believed for centuries that a vital, primordial, creative energy known as *kundalini*, or "coiled serpent power," lies dormant at the base of the spine. When aroused, this potential energy becomes activated. It rises up through a central channel in the body to unite with the power of cosmic consciousness that resides at the crown of the head, resulting in enlightenment and the release of tremendous amounts of creative energy. (See Chapter 7 for more information on the important role that kundalini plays in yoga philosophy.) A principal goal of yoga practices in general is to help awaken the dormant kundalini energy so that it may rise and lead to enlightenment. One way to help the kundalini awaken is to stoke the body with heat. Ashtanga Yoga is designed specifically to build up the internal heat in the body, particularly in the abdomen. This can contribute to the awakening of the kundalini energy.

Ashtanga Yoga: The Style

Ashtanga Yoga utilizes a prescribed series of sequential yoga postures. These postures, and the order in which they are performed, are especially designed to progressively heat, strengthen, and release the body. The series as a whole provides a complete workout for body, mind, and soul. Postures naturally complement one another to provide a precise balance of tightening and stretching. (For this reason, Ashtanga Yoga is sometimes referred to as "the hard and the soft" yoga.)

All postures within the Ashtanga Yoga sequence must be performed in the precise order in which they are prescribed to obtain the full benefit of this practice. Therefore, a session of Ashtanga Yoga always follows exactly the same format. There are, however, as many as six series of Ashtanga Yoga practice available—ranked by progressive difficulty—beginning with the Primary Series and moving on to more advanced ones.[5]

The first few series of Ashtanga Yoga are generally taught in a group class, although some men perform this practice on their own or under the guidance of a private teacher. As relatively few practitioners progress to the most difficult set of sequences, more advanced series are generally taught in individual sessions. It typically takes about 90 minutes to two hours to complete an Ashtanga Yoga practice series session.

A session of Ashtanga Yoga typically begins with an opening prayer, followed by a vigorous round of Sun Salutation exercises. (See the opening sequence of "A Complete Yoga Practice Session for Men," page 114.) The Salutations, which are performed with jumping movements, consist of several variations followed by a whole series of asanas. These postures, which include standing, seated, and inverted poses, provide a complete workout for the entire body. During the practice of the Sun Salutation and the asanas, practitioners employ ujjayi breathing, apply the bandhas, and fix the gaze on one of nine prescribed points of vision. A session of Ashtanga Yoga routinely ends with a closing series that includes stretching and relaxation.

As more yoga teachers study and incorporate the principles of Ashtanga Yoga into their practice, a wider variety of approaches to this flowing style are becoming increasingly more available. Because the original approach to the sequences may prove too demanding for some students, teachers are modifying the practice so as to maintain the flow and high energy level that accompanies it with easier and more comfortable postures. Often, they call their approach to yoga simply "Vinyasa Yoga," emphasizing the flowing quality of the sequences, but downplaying the "Power" aspect of the unadulterated Ashtanga Yoga practice. (See "Vinyasa Yoga," page 108.)

Ashtanga Yoga is proving itself very popular with men because of its vigorous physicality. Many people who are physically active or who are trying to recover from physical injury are attracted to the practice because of its emphasis on strength and endurance. Ashtanga Yoga can help to align, detoxify, and calm the body. While Ashtanga Yoga emphasizes physical strength and stamina, a man need not necessarily be strong and fit to practice this style of yoga. Indeed, the practice of Ashtanga Yoga can help make you fit and strong.

Ashtanga Yoga is a vigorous approach to the practice of yoga. It may not be suitable for all individuals—especially those with severe physical complaints or concerns. However, because the postures of the Ashtanga Yoga series can be modified to accommodate specific needs, you should be able to find a teacher who can help you benefit from Ashtanga Yoga. This style of yoga is specifically designed to help build strength and endurance and increase flexibility and range of motion. With appropriate instruction, Ashtanga Yoga may, in fact, appeal to some men who are trying to strengthen bodies weakened or compromised by illness or injury.

Background and Training of Practitioners

Because Ashtanga Yoga was "rediscovered" in India only within the last 75 years or so and introduced to the West even more recently than that, it is still a relatively new approach to yoga in the West. Unlike the other major styles of yoga that are associated with established institutes and training centers, there is no central organization that trains and certifies teachers of Ashtanga Yoga.

Because of its increasing popularity, however, you should have no trouble finding a teacher of Ashtanga, or Power, Yoga. In evaluating a prospective teacher of Ashtanga Yoga, be discriminating. Ashtanga Yoga is a physically challenging and demanding approach to yoga. The practices of which it is comprised, such as ujjayi breathing and the application of the yogic seals, can take many years of experience to perfect. In searching for a teacher of Ashtanga Yoga, as in any other style of yoga, check teachers' backgrounds carefully. Find out how long they have been studying this style of yoga, with whom they studied, and how regularly and actively they practice themselves. In addition, you might check with other people who have studied with a prospective teacher as well as sit in on or attend a single class before committing to a program of study with a particular teacher.

For Further Information

K. Pattabhi Jois founded the Ashtanga Yoga Research Institute in Mysore, India, which is the center for the teaching of his Ashtanga Yoga method. The Institute's Website contains detailed photographs of the postures that form the various series of Ashtanga Yoga. For further information on the Institute and Jois's method, classes, workshops, and worldwide teaching schedule, visit *www.ayri.org*.

Beryl Bender Birch is one of the most prominent spokespeople for Ashtanga Yoga in the United States. She and her husband, Thom, teach Ashtanga Yoga at yoga centers in New York City; East Hampton, New York; and elsewhere at a variety of learning retreats, yoga centers, and other venues. In addition, they train teachers in this style of yoga.

For further information on classes, programs, books, tapes, and other resources provided by Thom and Beryl Bender Birch, contact:

Power Yoga
The Hard & The Soft Astanga Yoga Institute
P.O. Box 1235
East Hampton, NY 11937
Tel: (212) 661-2895
Website: *www.power-yoga.com*
E-mail: yoga@power-yoga.com

Richard Freeman is one of the most preeminent teachers of Ashtanga Yoga. He teaches workshops around the country and has produced a variety of Ashtanga Yoga practice videos and DVDs. For further information on Richard Freeman and his classes and videos, contact:

The Yoga Workshop
2020 21st Street
Boulder, CO 80302
Website: *www.yogaworkshop.com*
E-mail: yogaworkshop@mindspring.com

Tim Miller was the first American to be certified as a teacher of yoga by K. Pattabhi Jois at the Ashtanga Yoga Research Institute in Mysore, India. For further information on his

Ashtanga Yoga Center in Encinitas, California, classes, and national and international teaching schedules, contact:

Ashtanga Yoga Center

118 West E Street

Encinitas, CA 92024

Tel: (760) 632-7093

Website: *www.ashtangayogacenter.com*

E-mail: ashtangayoga@cox.net

Go to *www.ashtanga.com* for additional information regarding Ashtanga Yoga, including a rich archive of articles on Ashtanga Yoga, a database of teachers searchable by geographic location, a list of classes and workshops in Ashtanga Yoga, and an extensive list of links to other Websites for additional information on Ashtanga Yoga.

Suggested Further Resources

Beryl Bender Birch, *Power Yoga: The Total Strength and Flexibility Workout* (Fireside, 1995). This is a leading text on Ashtanga Yoga, written by one of the foremost teachers and practitioners of this style of yoga. It includes an introduction to Ashtanga Yoga as well as complete instructions on how to practice Ashtanga Yoga. This reference is richly illustrated to show the exact position for each pose.

————, *Beyond Power Yoga: 8 Levels of Practice for Body and Soul* (Fireside, 2000). This book explores the complete classical Ashtanga Yoga system and discusses how it can be used to balance and heal body, mind, and soul.

Sri K. Pattabhi Jois, *Yoga Mala: The Seminal Treatise and Guide from the Living Master of Ashtanga Yoga,* 3rd edition (North Point Press, 2002). Jois presents the ethical principles and philosophy underlying his approach to yoga and guides the reader through the Sun Salutations and the Primary Series of Ashtanga Yoga, consisting of 42 asanas with precise instructions and descriptions of the benefits of each pose.

John Scott, *Ashtanga Yoga: The Definitive Step-by-Step Guide to Dynamic Yoga* (Crown, 2001). This easy-to-use guide draws on John Scott's expertise as a teacher of Ashtanga Yoga and features color photographs and a series of step-by-step exercise sessions to get you started on a simple sequence designed for beginners.

David Swenson, *Ashtanga Yoga: The Practice Manual: An Illustrated Guide to Personal Practice, The Primary & Intermediate Series plus Three Short Forms* (Ashtanga Yoga Productions, 1990). This spiral-bound practice guide contains complete instructions for the primary and intermediate Ashtanga Yoga series, as well as three shortened forms, complete with 650 illustrations. The author is one of the foremost instructors of Ashtanga Yoga in the United States, having studied with both David Williams and K. Pattabhi Jois. This book provides some of the best and most precise descriptions for performing Ashtanga Yoga postures.

Thom Birch on yoga for men:

"I was a track and field athlete from the time I was a child. I was nationally ranked as a runner at the age of 14. As little boys, we're taught to 'strengthen, strengthen, strengthen' and 'tighten, tighten, tighten.' It wasn't until I discovered yoga that I realized that we can become softer and more flexible to get strong. I found that yoga is an entire set of practices that can show us another side of life. Men can avail themselves of yoga to become soft and strong at the same time, and in the process discover a whole different side of themselves."

—Thom Birch, Teacher of Ashtanga Yoga at the New York Road Runners Club since 1986 and Musician/Songwriter who created the CD, *Chanting Soul*

Richard Freeman on yoga for men:

"Ashtanga practice can lead quickly into the subtle and delightful thread upon which all types of yoga move."

—Richard Freeman, Director of the Yoga Workshop in Boulder, Colorado, has studied Ashtanga Yoga with K. Pattabhi Jois and has produced a series of DVDs on Ashtanga Yoga practice

Chapter 7

KUNDALINI YOGA

Igniting the Fire Within

Suddenly, with a roar like that of a waterfall, I felt a stream of liquid light entering my brain through the spinal cord.

Entirely unprepared for such a development, I was completely taken by surprise; but regaining self-control instantaneously, I remained sitting in the same posture, keeping my mind on the point of concentration. The illumination grew brighter and brighter, the roaring louder, I experienced a rocking sensation and then felt myself slipping out of my body, entirely enveloped in a halo of light. It is impossible to describe the experience accurately.[1]

—Gopi Krishna

What Is Kundalini Yoga?

Kundalini (from *kundala*, or "coiled," in Sanskrit) yoga is an approach to yoga that emphasizes yoga's ability to release a powerful creative energy known in Sanskrit as *kundalini–shakti* ("female serpent power"). The kundalini energy is believed to lie dormant at the base of the spine, like a coiled snake. Through a variety of practices, including physical postures, special breathing techniques, mantra recitation, and meditation, practitioners of kundalini yoga strive to awaken this dormant energy. The awakening of the kundalini energy can help lead an individual to self-realization and enlightenment. Some practitioners translate *kundalini* as "the curl of the lock of hair of the beloved"—by uncoiling this lock of hair, we can unite our individual self with the consciousness of the universe.[2]

75

The Origins of Kundalini Yoga

The origins of kundalini yoga are obscure. Adding to the mystique surrounding kundalini yoga is that its practice has often been shrouded in secrecy, traditionally reserved for mystics and occult practitioners. However, references to the tremendous power associated with kundalini-shakti date back to some of the earliest known texts on yoga.

The kundalini represents a somewhat mysterious yet enormously powerful energy that is present both within the universe and within each individual. It is conceived of as the divine feminine principle upon which the universe is founded. Through the practice of kundalini yoga, the adept releases this energy so that it might rise up through the spine and be connected with the masculine energy, *shiva* ("benevolent") that is believed to reside at the crown of the head. The unification of the masculine and feminine energies in the body results in the highest union of yoga, leading to enlightenment, dissolution of the self, and realization of unbound bliss.

The *Yoga-Shikha-Upanishad* ("Secret Doctrine of the Crest of Yoga") is an ancient scripture that deals specifically with the process of raising the kundalini serpent power.[3] This text refers to kundalini yoga as the combined practice of mantra yoga, laya yoga, and hatha yoga. Kundalini yoga is also considered to participate in the tradition of tantra yoga. The asanas and breathing exercises that form a common base in hatha yoga are believed to purify and steady the body and mind for the tremendous outpouring of energy released by the rousing of the kundalini energy.

Kundalini (from *kundala*, or "coiled," in Sanskrit) yoga is an approach to yoga that emphasizes yoga's ability to release a powerful feminine, creative energy known in Sanskrit as *kundalini–shakti* ("female serpent power"). The kundalini energy is believed to lie dormant at the base of the spine, like a coiled snake. Through a variety of practices, including physical postures, special breathing techniques, mantra recitation, and meditation, practitioners of kundalini yoga strive to awaken this dormant energy. Once aroused, the kundalini energy ascends to the crown of the head, where it unites with *shiva*, the male principle of cosmic consciousness. The awakening of the kundalini energy and the union of feminine and masculine principles can help lead a man to self-realization and enlightenment.

Kundalini yoga was made prominent in recent history most notably through the dramatic experiences of Gopi Krishna (1903–1984.) An East Indian civil servant, Krishna practiced a type of yoga that was designed to unleash the kundalini serpent power. Despite his study and practice of this discipline, he was unprepared for the sheer power of the kundalini energy when it did finally rise within him. Krishna presented a vivid description of the tremendous psychoenergetic force that was unleashed in his autobiographical account, *Kundalini: The Evolutionary Energy in Man*. His book remains one of the most powerful firsthand accounts of kundalini ever written.

Kundalini yoga was made more widely available in the West primarily through the teachings of the East Indian master of kundalini yoga and spiritual teacher, Yogi Bhajan (1929–). All forms of yoga can raise the kundalini energy. Yogi Bhajan teaches kundalini yoga as a technology that allows one to maintain the energy and circulate it for maximum benefits. His approach also provides protection against some of the unpleasant experiences that some people seem to have had when their kundalini energy was spontaneously awakened. Yogi Bhajan first visited the United States in 1969, when he began to teach kundalini yoga and train teachers in his particular approach to yoga. Bhajan's work is carried on through the 3HO (Healthy, Happy, Holy) Foundation. Headquartered in New Mexico, 3HO is an international organization that promotes the practice of kundalini yoga throughout the world.

The Theory Underlying Kundalini Yoga

Kundalini yoga embraces the principle that we are more than just our physical bodies. In addition to the physical body, we have a number of other "bodies"—layers and sheaths that are normally imperceptible to the human eye. These subtle bodies overlay and interpenetrate one another. Sometimes referred to as etheric bodies, they are related to such areas as the emotional, mental, and spiritual aspects of ourselves. The yoga tradition maintains that contained within these bodies is also the blueprint for our entire development, present in the form of "seeds" that we brought forward into this life from past lives. One of the goals of yoga is to bring harmony to all the various aspects of the self that are contained within these various bodies.

Within the tradition of yoga lies a body of knowledge that might be referred to as the "Subtle Anatomy of Yoga." According to this esoteric anatomy, we are animated by a virtually countless number of vessels and channels that supply energy to all of our bodies. In the physical body, these vessels and channels are the blood vessels, nerve passageways, and other anatomical conduits that are known to medical science. On a more subtle level, we possess a nearly countless number of channels through which vital life energy, or prana, flows. These channels are called *nadis* ("channels"). Various authorities estimate these channels to be at different numbers. Most traditional sources maintain that there are 72,000 nadis in all, while some others maintain that there are several hundred thousand or more—even as many as billions.[4] In any case, it is easy to see that the nadis are virtually infinite, taxing the ability of the mind to map or to envision them in their totality.

Within this anatomy of man's subtle being, there are certain channels and confluences of nadis that are particularly important. Three channels that run along the spine form the most important passageways of energy in the body. These are the *sushumna* ("most gracious"), *ida* ("comfort"), and *pingala* ("tawny") nadis. The sushumna is the central of these three nadis, running from the base of the spine to the crown of the head. It is the channel through which the kundalini energy flows. Running alongside and spiraling around the sushumna so that they intersect one another at key points lie the ida and pingala nadis. The ida nadi begins at the base of the spine, where it flows along the left side of the body, coils around the central sushumna nadi, and terminates in the left nostril. The pingala nadi originates at the base of the spine, where it flows along the right side of the body, coils around the central sushumna nadi, and terminates in the right nostril. The ida and pingala channels represent feminine and masculine energy, respectively.

In the average person, unawakened to the energy of kundalini-shakti, energy flows only through the two side channels, ida and pingala. The energy is believed to flow alternately through each of these two channels for periods of roughly one hour and 45 minutes to two hours at a time, during which period the breath through one nostril is dominant.[5] This creates a rhythmic flow of energy through the body. One of the goals of the practice of pranayama, or breath control, is to help balance and regulate the flow of energy through these two channels. The goal of kundalini yoga is to awaken the kundalini serpent energy that lies coiled at the base of the spine so that it might rise up through sushumna, resulting in enlightenment.

Along the midline of the body at strategic points lie a series of psychoenergetic centers known as chakras (cakra, "wheel" or "circle" in Sanskrit). The chakras lie at the points where ida and pingala intersect one another as they coil around sushumna. Other nadis also converge at the chakras, so that the chakras might be likened to ganglia or plexuses of subtle energy channels. The chakras are frequently compared to energy transformers: They take in the vital energy of prana from the atmosphere around us and transform it so that it can be circulated throughout and used by both the physical and subtle bodies. According to many authoritative sources, there are seven major chakras that lie along the midline of the body and progress from the base of the spine to the crown of the head.[6]

The first chakra, muladhara ("foundation" or "root support" in Sanskrit), commonly referred to as the root chakra, originates at the base of the spine. The root chakra is concerned with our physical vitality and survival. The second chakra, svadhisthana ("dwelling place of the self"), commonly referred to as either the sacral or the sexual chakra, is situated in the pelvic bowl, about two inches below the navel. The second chakra is associated with our sexuality and connection to other people. The third chakra, manipura ("the city of gems"), referred to as the solar plexus chakra, is situated in the solar plexus. This chakra is associated with our sense of self-esteem and power. The fourth chakra, anahata ("unstruck sound"), or the heart chakra, is located in the center of the breast between the two nipples—an area frequently referred to as the heart center. The heart chakra is associated with love and compassion. The fifth chakra, vishuddha ("pure"), or the throat chakra, is situated in the hollow in the center of the throat. This chakra is associated with communication and creativity. The sixth chakra, ajna ("command" or "authority"), known as the brow or third-eye chakra, is situated deep in the center of the head at a level between the two eyebrows. The sixth chakra is associated with intuition and our ability to communicate mind-to-mind with other beings and the spirit world. The seventh chakra is the last chakra. It is known as sahasrara ("thousand-petaled"), or the crown chakra, and is located at or just above the crown of the head. The crown chakra is associated with our connection to universal spirit, the source of our being.

The seventh chakra is referred to metaphorically as the "thousand-petaled lotus." It is the highest of the chakras. When the kundalini energy rises up through the central sushumna channel, the kundalini fully activates, charges, and harmonizes all of the chakras in the body in its upward ascent. The feminine energy of kundalini-shakti stored at the base of the spine finds union with shiva, the masculine principle of consciousness. When this occurs, a man achieves self-realization and enlightenment.

A primary goal of many yoga practices is to prepare the practitioner for the flow of kundalini energy up through the spine and the important energy centers that lie along it. This is why many physical yoga postures are designed to support optimum strength, flexibility, and stability of the spine.

The following illustration depicts schematically the pathways of the three central channels of energy and the location of the seven major chakras that lie along the spine:

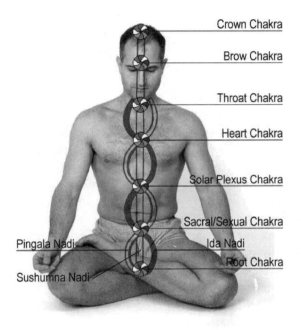

Fig. 7.1: Yoga Subtle Anatomy—the Chakras and Central Energy Channels

The kundalini energy lies coiled at the base of the spine, like a cobra. For this reason, it is sometimes referred to as the serpent power. It is the primeval energy of the universe and a bridge of transformation from the self to the infinite. Some authorities maintain that kundalini-shakti lies coiled three and one-half times with its head facing downward. Others claim that it lies coiled as many as eight and one-half times. Whatever the number of coils, the purpose of kundalini yoga is to release the energy that is contained in the coiled serpent power. Uncoiled, the head of kundalini-shakti races upward, like the head of an uncoiling cobra, and finds union with the thousand-petaled lotus at the seventh, or crown, chakra. In the process of this upward rising, kundalini-shakti can give off tremendous energy in the form of heat and light. This movement of kundalini is often compared to a variety of phenomena, such as a streak of lightning or the release of an intense stream of steam.

Kundalini Yoga: The Style

Kundalini yoga draws on time-honored practices to prepare and encourage the kundalini energy to rise. It is believed that heat contributes to the arousal of the kundalini. Some of the techniques that are used in kundalini yoga are aimed specifically to increase the heat in the body. Thus, relatively active physical movements can be used. These can include traditional asanas that are performed with more vigor and motion than typical hatha yoga practices. For instance, the Sun Salutation series (see page 114) might be performed with jumps included. The Bridge Pose (see Fig. YPS.11 on page 131) might be made more active by the practitioner alternately bending and straightening the arms to raise and lower the back, torso, and core of the body up and down in a rhythmic pumping motion. In addition, physical movements that involve twisting and moving the spine vigorously can help activate the energy in the spine. The application of locks and seals (for instance, contracting the area of the anal sphincter or planting the tongue against the roof of the mouth) can be used to seal in as much energy as possible so that it remains contained and is not dissipated. The use of specific yogic breathing techniques can be used to build up additional internal heat. The recitation of special sacred mantras and meditation on such objects as the chakras can further add to the building up of heat and energy in the body.

All of these techniques taken together create what might be likened to a combustion chamber in which kundalini energy is ignited and released. The techniques that are used in kundalini yoga are designed not only to foster the release of kundalini-shakti, but also to strengthen and stabilize the body so that it will be prepared for the powerful onslaught of kundalini energy when it is eventually released. Aside from the preparation for handling the release of kundalini energy, these practices have overall positive effects, such as strengthening the body and mind, promoting harmony and balance, and purifying the body of toxins, including not only physical waste products, but also emotional and mental debris.

Kundalini yoga holds special appeal for any man trying to explore the psychospiritual aspect of himself. The practice of kundalini yoga participates in age-old rites designed to raise the individual's level of energy to merge with the primordial feminine creative urge that gave rise to the creation of the universe. When kundalini energy is released in this way, a man can attain the ultimate goal of yoga: the ecstatic bliss of oneness with all being.

Kundalini yoga can also be distinctively fun. All yoga postures can be performed with a playful spontaneity. Kundalini yoga, in particular, however, often employs rolling, rocking, and twisting movements that can be especially physically enjoyable to do. This particular style of yoga reminds us that yoga developed initially as a vibrant, lived experience. The physical asanas were discovered naturally and spontaneously by intuitive seekers who were in tune with their own bodies and incorporated natural movements into the practice of yoga. It is only over time that yoga has become compartmentalized and subdivided into all the various branches and systems that tend to emphasize specific aspects of it.

Kundalini yoga attempts to raise a very powerful force of energy. The rush of energy that can be involved in kundalini could be overwhelming and disorienting to someone who is not adequately prepared for it. For this reason, the practice of kundalini yoga is best pursued under the guidance of a teacher who has great depth of experience, and who can help you develop adequate physical, mental, and emotional stability in your practice.

In individuals who are not adequately prepared for the uprising of kundalini energy, or who are psychologically unstable, the accidental rising of kundalini could lead to nervous disorders, including psychotic episodes. A number of associations and support networks have been established to help individuals in crisis from a kundalini experience cope with the effects of spontaneous, premature, or unprepared episodes of kundalini uprisings (see page 82). A number of psychiatrists and experts in the field of spiritual development, notably Dr. Stanislav Grof, M.D., and his wife Christina, have observed that in some cases, individuals who are in the process of spiritual "emergency" (that is, for whom spirit is emerging) are diagnosed as being mentally ill. The Suggested Further Reading section at the end of this chapter contains titles of books that are of particular interest in this regard.

Background and Training of Practitioners

Many of the teachers of kundalini yoga in the West today have been trained, directly or indirectly, by Yogi Bhajan and the 3HO Foundation he established in 1969. Training requires extensive experience in the practice of kundalini yoga as well as intensive retreats.

For further information on kundalini yoga as taught by Yogi Bhajan and his 3HO Foundation, contact:

3HO International Headquarters

P.O. Box 2337

Espanola, NM 87532

Tel: (888) 346-2420 or (505) 753-4988

Fax: (505) 753-1999

Website: *www.3ho.org*

E-mail: yogainfo@3ho.org

You can also find valuable information on kundalini yoga, including a list of kundalini yoga teachers and teacher training programs from the International Kundalini Yoga Teacher's Association (IKYTA):

3HO IKYTA

3 Ram Das Guru Place

Espanola, NM 87532

Tel: (505) 753-0423

Fax: (505) 753-5982

Website: *www.kundaliniyoga.com*

E-mail: ikyta@3ho.org (customer service)

For Further Information

In addition to the resources cited previously, Ravi Singh is a prominent presenter of an approach to kundalini yoga. He teaches ongoing classes in New York City and workshops worldwide. For current information regarding Ravi Singh's schedule, as well as his books and tapes, contact:

Ravi Singh

Tel: (800) 243-YOGA

Website: *www.raviyoga.com*

E-mail: raviyoga@aol.com

For those individuals in a state of spiritual emergency, two organizations can be of assistance:

The Center for Psychological & Spiritual Health (CPSH) was founded in 1980 as the Spiritual Emergency Network by Christina Grof and her husband, Stanislav Grof. The CPSH provides information, referrals, and support for individuals experiencing spiritual emergence and difficulty in psychospiritual growth, either through the experience of kundalini uprisings or other precipitating factors. For further information:

Center for Psychological & Spiritual Health

1453 Mission Street

San Francisco, CA 94103

Tel: (415) 575-6299

Website: *www.cpsh.org/*

E-mail: cpsh@ciis.edu

The Kundalini Clinic for Counseling and Research is the first spiritual emergence service in the world, founded in 1976 by Lee Sannella, M.D., author of *The Kundalini Experience*. It is directed by Stuart Sovatsky, Ph.D., author of *Words from the Soul*. The clinic provides technical information on yogic approaches to difficulties sometimes experienced with kundalini activity and also weekly therapy sessions to help people integrate such awakenings into their daily lives, careers, and relationships—locally in person or nationally and internationally by phone. For further information:

The Kundalini Clinic

3040 Richmond Boulevard

Oakland, CA 94611

Tel: (510) 232-8262

Website: *home.jps.net/~stuartcs*

E-mail:stuartcs@jps.net

Suggested Further Reading

The following books are on kundalini yoga and the chakras:

Gopi Krishna *Kundalini: The Evolutionary Energy in Man* (Shambhala, 1985). This is a riveting autobiographical account of kundalini yoga by one of the modern era's most celebrated kundalini yogis.

Shakta Kaur Khalsa *Kundalini YogaKundalini Yoga: Unlock Your Inner Potential Through Life-Changing Practices* (DK Publishing, 2001). This is a complete illustrated guide to the full range of kundalini yoga practices as taught by Yogi Bhajan, presenting them in a simple, easy-to-follow approach.

Shakti Parwha Kaur Khalsa, *Kundalini Yoga: The Flow of Eternal Power: A Simple Guide to the Yoga of Awareness* (Perigee, 1996). Written by one of Yogi Bhajan's students, this book is more a guide to the kundalini yoga principles and philosophy than to the physical practices.

Swami Sivananda Radha *Kundalini Yoga for the West: A Foundation for Character Building, Courage and Awareness* (Timeless Books, 1978). Swami Sivananda Radha, born in Germany and the first Western woman to become a swami, trained under the tutelage of Swami Sivananda. This book is an excellent introduction to kundalini yoga, tying it into the practice of yoga in general and elaborating on the psychological and moral aspects of this practice. (For more information on Swami Radha, see the entry for "Hidden Language of Hatha Yoga" on page102.)

Ravi Singh, *Kundalini Yoga for Body, Mind and Beyond* (White Lion Press, 2002). Written by a well-known presenter of kundalini yoga, this book is good for people starting or deepening their kundalini yoga practice. Of particular interest to male readers, it includes a chapter called "Manpower," which addresses men's issues, and another chapter called "Beyond Sex Together," which presents couples' exercises that relate to the issues of sex and relationships.

Susan G. Shumsky, *Exploring Chakras: Awaken Your Untapped Energy* (New Page Books, 2003). A seeker of esoteric truth for more than 35 years, the author distills the essence of the teachings of kundalini energy and the chakra system into a highly readable and comprehensive overview of the subtle anatomy of yoga and human energy.

The following books address the subject of spiritual emergency:

Christina Grof, and Stanislav Grof, M.D. *The Stormy Search for the Self: A Guide to Personal Growth Through Transformational Crisis* (J.P. Tarcher, 1990).

Stanislav Grof, M.D., and Christina Grof, *Spiritual Emergency: When Personal Transformation Becomes a Crisis* (J.P. Tarcher, 1989).

Ravi Singh on yoga for men:

"Yoga, especially kundalini yoga, offers sophisticated approaches to enhance every aspect of a man's health, relationships, career, and inner life. Men can benefit through kundalini yoga's ability to strengthen the nervous system, detoxify, increase flexibility, and help work through emotional armoring in the body. It also increases potency, mental focus, and makes one fearless. A man should be a warrior and poet, lover and provider. Kundalini yoga can help one embrace and embody these polarities."

—Ravi Singh, Author of *Kundalini Yoga for Body, Mind, and Beyond*

PART III

CONTEMPORARY ADAPTATIONS OF YOGA

The roots of yoga go back thousands of years to ancient India. However, yoga is a living and dynamic system of practice. It continues to grow and develop. As Westerners embrace the practice of yoga, they are integrating the experience they have gained in the main styles of traditional yoga practice with their own personal experiences. Following the first wave of yoga teachers who helped establish the main traditions of yoga practice in the West, a new crop of yoga teachers is helping to redefine yoga practice today. These teachers are developing their own integrative approaches to yoga, taking into account the needs of modern Western men. Many of the new innovators are Westerners, primarily American. Emerging approaches to yoga that combine the best of East and West, ancient and modern wisdom, are now being introduced and practiced throughout the United States.

The following chapters introduce some of the most widely practiced and innovative of the emerging approaches to yoga that you're likely to encounter on your own individual yoga journey. In Chapter 10, you'll also find descriptions of several more traditional approaches that you may come across in your yoga journey. Following the chapters in this section, you'll find a section titled "A Complete Yoga Practice Session for Men" that incorporates the foundational elements that underlie many styles of yoga practiced today.

Chapter 8

KRIPALU YOGA

Breath, Meditation, and Motion

Kripalu Yoga is a powerful, transformational practice that integrates all the parts of who you are. It's a clearing process, a way of encountering and releasing physical, mental, and emotional blocks.[1]

—The Kripalu Experience

What Is Kripalu Yoga?

Kripalu (pronounced Krih-PAH-loo) means "being compassionate" in Sanskrit. Kripalu Yoga is a contemporary, integrative approach to yoga that synthesizes traditional Eastern yoga practices with the unique needs of contemporary men living an active lifestyle. It also integrates Western psychological insights into the practice of yoga. This style of yoga aims to help each individual discover and release physical, mental, and emotional blockages. Kripalu Yoga was developed and continues to evolve as a collaborative effort of the members of the Kripalu Center for Yoga and Health (Kripalu Center), a spiritual fellowship community in Lenox, in the Berkshire Hills of Massachusetts.

The Origins of Kripalu Yoga

Kripalu Yoga is inspired by the life and teachings of the Indian spiritual master Swami Kripalu (1913–1981). Revered in India for his love of God, service to humanity, and mastery of yoga, Swami Kripalu was an accomplished scholar and musician who maintained a rigorous schedule of 10 hours of intensive spiritual practice per day. Through the disciplines of yoga, he awakened the latent life force energy of prana and kundalini within

Kripalu (pronounced Krih-PAH-loo) means "being compassionate" in Sanskrit. Kripalu Yoga is a contemporary, integrative approach to yoga that synthesizes traditional Eastern yoga practices with the unique needs of contemporary men living active lifestyles. It also integrates Western psychological insights into the practice of yoga. Kripalu Yoga aims to help each individual discover and release physical, mental, and emotional blockages.

Kripalu Yoga was developed as a collaborative effort of the members of the Kripalu Center, a spiritual fellowship community located in Lenox, Massachusetts. The Kripalu Center was originally founded by followers of the revered Indian spiritual teacher Swami Kripalu (1913–1981) and, in particular, his student Yogi Amrit Desai. Since Yogi Desai's departure from the Kripalu Center in 1994, Kripalu's unique approach to living continues to evolve as The Kripalu Approach to Health, Growth, and Transformation. Kripalu Yoga is practiced throughout the United States and the world by the many thousands of students and teachers who have been trained in this approach to yoga.

his body. His teachings flowed from a rich reservoir of personal spiritual experience.

Yogi Amrit Desai, a close disciple of Swami Kripalu, came to America in 1960 to study art and teach yoga. In 1970, Yogi Desai had a profound yoga experience that led him to adapt Swami Kripalu's traditional teachings into a format suited to the needs of active Westerners. He called this approach Kripalu Yoga. Kripalu Yoga is unique in that it teaches a practitioner how to activate prana and harness this life force energy for healing and spiritual growth.

Yogi Desai founded the original Kripalu Center in 1974 in Pennsylvania. In 1977, Swami Kripalu traveled to America to reside at the Kripalu Center, where he stayed for four years. Swami Kripalu was directly involved in the development of Kripalu Yoga. In 1981, Swami Kripalu returned to India, where he died shortly after his return. In 1984, the Kripalu Center was relocated to its current location in the Berkshires.

For more than 20 years, Yogi Desai worked with many gifted Kripalu residents to integrate Western principles of holistic health and psychology with the traditional Eastern approach to yoga. Since Yogi Desai's departure from the Kripalu Center in 1994, Kripalu's unique approach to living continues to evolve as The Kripalu Approach to Health, Growth, and Transformation.

Kripalu Yoga continues to be taught at the Kripalu Center and by certified teachers throughout the world. In addition to a dizzying array of yoga classes and workshop programs, the Center offers frequent teacher training programs in its approach to yoga, certifying thousands of teachers in various levels of practice of Kripalu Yoga.

The Theory Underlying Kripalu Yoga

Kripalu Yoga is based on the yogic belief that body, mind, and spirit are connected by the flow of an intelligent life force called prana. Attuning to this energy not only enhances health, but it also stimulates psychological growth and spiritual awakening. Kripalu Yoga utilizes a wide variety of techniques, including asana practice, meditation, breathing techniques, and the principles of a yoga lifestyle to promote inner harmony and self-transformation.

Kripalu Yoga is comprised of three levels of practice. In the first level, Stage One, known as "willful practice," students learn how to practice the classic postures of hatha yoga with relaxation, deep breathing, and proper alignment. Poses are held for a relatively short period of time—generally three to five flowing breaths (approximately 10 to 20 seconds). Stage One practice strengthens the body, releases chronic tension, engenders an attitude of compassionate self-acceptance, and helps prepare practitioners for deeper practice.

In Stage Two, postures are held for a longer period of time to foster an inner balance of "will and surrender." The purpose of Stage Two practice is to become attuned to the presence and flow of prana. Holding poses for a prolonged period of time allows practitioners to focus attention inward. The mind is focused on the sensations, emotions, and thoughts that arise during holding and the body is moved in slow motion as guided from within. An ability to closely observe the interplay of body and mind, which is called witness consciousness, is acquired. Stage Two practice helps bring practitioners from a place of what is known and comfortable to one that is uncomfortable. At this pivotal point, fears and resistances emerge. Confronting physical, mental, and emotional fear and resistance can be a path to releasing blocked energies. Clearing blockages can be a tremendously therapeutic process on the path of self-transformation.

In Stage Three, "surrender to the wisdom of the body," prana grows stronger and the ability of the mind to witness its activity increases. The practitioner offers his body to Spirit and invites prana to be the guide, allowing the wisdom of the body to emerge spontaneously. Practitioners are guided by the body's innate knowing to enter traditional yoga postures or create totally new ways of being. Yoga thus becomes a meditation in motion directed by the flow of prana as it courses through the body-mind. Kripalu's approach recognizes that the essence of meditation is a state of inner absorption that can occur in either the flow of movement or moments of physical stillness. Both meditation-in-motion and sitting meditation are seen as valid and complementary practices.

The Kripalu Center has served as a location that has attracted many practitioners of yoga who have desired to share their knowledge of yoga and grow in their practice of yoga through collaboration with others. The Kripalu Center regularly sponsors conferences with titles such as "Yoga at the Leading Edge," "Yoga and Buddhism," and "Psychotherapy and Spirituality" that gather together in one location at one time some of the most well-known teachers of a wide variety of yoga styles.

Through the collaborative efforts of its residents, teachers, and directors, many innovative adaptations and approaches to yoga have developed that combine talk, assisted partnering, movement and dance, and partner massage. One major style of yoga that emerged as a result of the experience of Kripalu Yoga is Michael Lee's pioneering Phoenix Rising Yoga Therapy. This approach to yoga has become so rich and widely practiced that it is treated in depth in the following chapter.

Kripalu Yoga: The Style

Kripalu Yoga is most commonly practiced in a class setting, although individual instruction by certified Kripalu Yoga teachers is also available, in Lenox and in many other locations. Classes are approximately one hour to two hours in length. They incorporate exercise of physical postures, focused awareness on the breath, and motion. Classes can be grouped according to the three levels of practice, although "open" classes geared for anyone at any level are also widely available. The amount of physical exertion used can range from gentle to intense. Generally, the emphasis in Kripalu Yoga is on precision of form and awareness, rather than physical effort.

Kripalu Yoga can be especially beneficial to those individuals seeking to combine the practice of yoga with personal transformation. By engaging himself fully in the practice of Kripalu Yoga and bringing the focus and attention to every detail of the physical postures, a man can relax the body, calm the mind, and strengthen one's self from within. Perhaps more importantly, Kripalu Yoga emphasizes letting go of emotional blocks and regaining the ability to feel fully. This can bring a man back in touch with his feelings, often opening his heart to himself and others. From this place of self-acceptance and emotional connection, the answers to life's questions become clearer and men can enjoy the bliss and inner freedom that is the goal of yoga. The Kripalu Center offers an ongoing assortment of programs that may be of particular interest to men, including workshops in yoga for back care and yoga for men.

Background and Training of Practitioners

Certification in Kripalu Yoga is provided through a training program offered at the Kripalu Center in Lenox, Massachusetts. Training programs are offered regularly throughout the year. The Basic Certification program requires intensive residential training. This training can be accomplished either in one full month of training or in a series of three nine-day residential training sessions spaced over a period of about six months. The Basic Certification program prepares individuals to teach Stage One postures. It teaches a detailed understanding of the asanas and pranayama (yogic breathing practices), including benefits and contraindications; anatomy and physiology as it relates to yoga practice; relaxation and meditation methodology; and the history and principles of yoga philosophy. Students practice teaching under supervision. Additional levels of training provide instruction in Stages Two and Three of Kripalu Yoga. It is recommended that candidates for Basic Certification training have at least six months' experience in daily practice of Kripalu Yoga. More than 5,000 teachers of Kripalu Yoga have been certified and are practicing throughout the world today.

For further information on Kripalu Yoga teacher training, contact:

Kripalu Center for Yoga and Health
P.O. Box 793
West Street, Route 183
Lenox, MA 01240
Tel: (800) 741-SELF or (413) 448-3152 (international and local calls)
Fax: (413) 448-3384
Website: *www.kripalu.org*
E-mail: request@kripalu.org (for general questions or to request a catalog)

For Further Information

The Kripalu Center is a nonprofit spiritual community that offers a wide range of courses and workshops in yoga and topics of associated interest. It has established itself as a preeminent alternative learning center, one of a growing network of such learning centers emerging around the world (see Chapter 17). The Kripalu Center offers a wide range of yoga programs, including yoga and cross-country skiing, yoga and biking, yoga for back care, "hot" yoga practiced in rooms heated to temperatures as high as 90 degrees Fahrenheit, and many more. Programs are offered in the Center's residential setting in the Berkshires. Accommodations and vegetarian food are available, as well as twice-daily classes in Kripalu Yoga. For further information on the Kripalu Center and to make reservations or appointments for private sessions, contact the Center according to the previously provided information. The Center's Website contains not only information on Kripalu, its programs, and teachers, but also a list of links to other useful yoga Websites. Currently, there are 24 Kripalu Yoga studios scattered around the country that can be easily located because the Website offers a "find a Kripalu Yoga Teacher or Affiliated Studio near you" service.

The Kripalu Yoga Teachers Association (KYTA) is the professional association of teachers of Kripalu Yoga. It can help you find a teacher of Kripalu Yoga or a class at an affiliated studio through its searchable database. For further information, contact:

Kripalu Yoga Teachers Association (KYTA)

Tel: (413) 448-3202

Website: *www.kripalu.org/yogateachers.html*

E-mail: kyta@kripalu.org

Suggested Further Resources

The staff of the Kripalu Center has created a variety of books, as well as audio- and videotapes on Kripalu Yoga. *Kripalu Hatha Yoga* by Christopher Ken Baxter presents 26 asanas accompanied by more than 125 illustrations that can help guide you through a complete and well-balanced hatha yoga routine. Videotapes include *Kripalu Yoga Gentle*, *Kripalu Yoga Dynamic*, and *Kripalu Yoga Partner*. Senior teacher Yogananda (Michael Carroll) has produced two compact discs on *pranayama*, featuring the Kripalu approach to yogic breathing at beginning and intermediate levels of practice. The Kripalu Center's audiocassettes present a number of different yoga sequences, and its music CDs can provide a relaxing accompaniment to your yoga routine. All of these items, plus additional titles, props, and accessories to assist you in your practice are available from the Center's bookshop, which can be reached by contacting the Kripalu Center or visiting its Website. In addition, as of the publication of this book, the first book devoted to Kripalu Yoga, *Kripalu Yoga: A Guide to Practice On and Off the Mat* by Richard Faulds, is scheduled for release by Bantam Books.

Richard Faulds on yoga for men:

"Although it can be practiced quite vigorously, Kripalu Yoga is not designed to be a 'killer workout.' It's a practice that enhances health, helps get you back in touch with your feelings and focuses the mind. Practiced regularly, Kripalu Yoga initiates a transformative process that opens the heart and expands awareness.

"The big issue for myself and many men is staying intimate with what we are feeling. Even the word 'intimate' used in reference to one's self pushes buttons in the male gender role. Life's very real challenges have led so many men to lose touch with their bodies, shut down emotionally, and get stuck in rigid ways of thinking and being.

"Because it is so effective at bringing a man back in touch with himself, Kripalu Yoga can be an extremely powerful practice for those men wanting to awaken to deeper levels of their being. Yoga can break the shell of alienation from the self and help a man regain sensitivity and emotional balance. This is not an easy process; it's the hero's journey into the face of fear and feeling through the body. The end result is a man that is strong *and* sensitive. This has been my experience, and that of many other men I have known."

—Richard Faulds, Senior Kripalu Yoga Teacher and Author of *Kripalu Yoga:*
A Guide to Practice On and Off the Mat

Chapter 9

PHOENIX RISING YOGA THERAPY

Yoga Therapy Meets Talk Therapy

I believe we can use our body as our teacher to access our inner wisdom ... Phoenix Rising Yoga Therapy is a practice that promotes transformation by drawing on the unique wisdom of the body.... When this happens, yoga is therapy.[1]

—Michael Lee

What Is Phoenix Rising Yoga Therapy?

Phoenix Rising Yoga Therapy is a contemporary approach to yoga that draws on the innate wisdom of the body to access the soul. Australian-born Michael Lee developed this approach to body/mind integration as a result of his own experience and practice of yoga and the yogic life. Phoenix Rising Yoga Therapy uses a variety of techniques, including assisted postures, breathing, non-directive dialogue, imagery, and meditation to foster inner awareness. The reference to the mythical phoenix in the name of this yoga therapy highlights its ability to be a powerful tool for personal growth and transformation.

The Origins of Phoenix Rising Yoga Therapy

Phoenix Rising Yoga Therapy is an emerging form of body/mind integration. It represents a synthesis of ancient yoga practices and modern insights into personal growth.

Michael Lee developed Phoenix Rising Yoga Therapy as a result of his unique life experiences. Lee, who was born in Adelaide, Australia, was trained in education and psychology and worked for a time as an organizational consultant to the Australian government.

Phoenix Rising Yoga Therapy is a contemporary approach to yoga that draws on the innate wisdom of the body to access the soul. Australian-born Michael Lee developed this approach to body/mind integration as a result of his own experience and practice of yoga and the yogic life. Phoenix Rising Yoga Therapy uses a variety of techniques, including assisted postures, breathing, non-directive dialogue, and meditation to foster inner awareness. The reference to the mythical phoenix in the name of this yoga therapy highlights its ability to be a powerful tool for personal growth and transformation.

Akin to many men today, he is also a spiritual seeker. His search for his own inner self led him to the practice of yoga. He experimented with a variety of approaches to yoga that eventually led him in the mid-1980s to become a resident at the Kripalu Center, where he learned, practiced, and taught that particular approach to yoga (see Chapter 8).

In practicing yoga, Lee became aware of its rich potential to be a tool for personal transformation. This became especially apparent to him when he practiced asana postures with the assistance of another man, who also served a mirroring function through his provision of interactive dialogue. Lee realized that when the practice of yoga postures was combined with the nurturing hands-on and verbal support of another sensitive, trained individual, a true therapy developed.

Lee created Phoenix Rising Yoga Therapy from these basic tools, and in 1986 established a private practice outside of ashram life. In 1987, he began to offer training workshops and certification programs to teach others his innovative, integrative approach to yoga. Since that time, Phoenix Rising Yoga Therapy has been practiced and taught throughout the United States, Canada, and Europe.

The Theory Underlying Phoenix Rising Yoga Therapy

Phoenix Rising Yoga Therapy is based on the belief that a man's body can be a rich reservoir of inner wisdom, which is a commonality among yogic principles in general and many other approaches to body/mind integration, both ancient and contemporary. Long after we have forgotten experiences and feelings in conscious awareness, the body remembers. By tapping into the wisdom of the body, men can bring to present awareness various issues that may have been limiting them, release those issues, and transform themselves. Phoenix Rising Yoga Therapy aims to provide a bridge from a man's body to his soul.

From personal experience, Lee discovered that the practice of yoga asanas, or postures, could guide us to greater presence in our bodies. This presence can lead us to the awareness that is necessary for integrating body and mind. Awareness is heightened when we practice yoga at what Lee describes as "the edge"—that point in a yoga posture at which any more stretch would be too much, and any less would not be enough. It is at this point that inner wisdom surfaces most profoundly.

Finding one's edge is a simple concept, but not necessarily easy to execute. Lee discovered that working with another person who provides both hands-on and non-directional, non-judgmental verbal assistance could help one find, maintain, and explore one's edge much more deeply. In addition to sharing insights, the partner provides the nurturing support of a caring and compassionate fellow human being. Through the postures, aware breathing, assisted support, and meditation, men who practice Phoenix Rising Yoga Therapy are able to achieve deep levels of awareness and acceptance of themselves as they are. This can be the first and key step in initiating a process of change to become who we truly are.

Phoenix Rising Yoga Therapy: The Style

Phoenix Rising Yoga Therapy is generally practiced in a one-on-one setting, with a trained practitioner assisting a client. Lee has trained many individuals in his style of yoga therapy throughout the world, and they are certified as practitioners to provide private sessions. Phoenix Rising Yoga Therapy can initiate a process of unfoldment, much like psychotherapy. For this reason, it can be helpful for a man to receive a number of ongoing sessions to explore various issues as they emerge. The number of sessions that might be helpful would, of course, depend upon each individual man's situation.

In addition to private sessions, workshops in Phoenix Rising Yoga Therapy are offered throughout the country at various learning networks and centers. These workshops can provide an opportunity to experience Phoenix Rising Yoga Therapy in a group setting with the support of a number of other people and for a more extended period of time.

Finally, a number of workshops and trainings are offered as part of the Phoenix Rising Yoga Therapy Certification Program. This program, which is open to anyone with some experience in yoga or another body/mind discipline, comprises various levels of training that provide direct, hands-on experience in the physical postures used in Phoenix Rising Yoga Therapy, as well as practice and guidance in verbal dialogue.

Phoenix Rising Yoga Therapy can be especially beneficial to those men seeking to combine their practice of yoga with greater in-depth exploration of the self. While many practitioners and teachers of yoga would agree that the goal of yoga is union of the body and mind, many specific styles of yoga focus on a particular aspect of yoga, such as the physical postures, breathing exercises, or meditation. Phoenix Rising Yoga Therapy consciously aims to integrate body, mind, and spirit through a rich synthesis of traditional and contemporary healing practices.

Phoenix Rising Yoga Therapy can provide men with many physical benefits; the assisted postures can help them go even more deeply into a pose than they would otherwise be able to on their own. This can help men take their practice of the asanas to a deeper level, in a safe and supportive environment. The benefits of a stronger and more healthful body can result. Phoenix Rising Yoga Therapy has been used by family therapists to help individuals recovering from substance abuse and to help clients dealing with emotional and physical issues following an injury or surgery. Phoenix Rising Yoga Therapy has also been used in programs of chronic pain management, smoking cessation, weight loss, stress-reduction, and for hyperactive and handicapped children.[2]

Phoenix Rising Yoga Therapy can also be extremely helpful for promoting a man's mental, psychological, and spiritual wellness. Through the practice of Phoenix Rising Yoga

Therapy, men can gain much greater clarity as mental, emotional, and psychological issues that may be providing a barrier to greater wholeness are resolved. In this regard, Phoenix Rising Yoga Therapy may be especially attractive as an adjunct to traditional psychotherapy or for men already engaged in other body/mind integration practices.

The practice of Phoenix Rising Yoga Therapy can result in bringing unconscious feelings, emotions, and attitudes to awareness. Therefore, it is best explored by those men having the mental and emotional stability to deal with any issues that emerge. Depending on the nature of issues that arise, it may be helpful for a man to seek appropriate psychological counseling in conjunction with Phoenix Rising Yoga Therapy. Certain postures may be contraindicated for individuals who underwent recent surgery or who have particular injuries.

Background and Training of Practitioners

Certification in Phoenix Rising Yoga Therapy is provided through the Phoenix Rising Yoga Therapy Professional Certification Training Program, which was designed by Michael Lee. Since the first practitioner trainings were offered in 1987, nearly 1,000 practitioners of Phoenix Rising Yoga Therapy have been certified and are practicing in virtually every state in the United States and in many foreign countries.

Certification in Phoenix Rising Yoga Therapy requires completion of three levels of training. Level I consists of a four-day intensive residential workshop that introduces the principles and practice of Phoenix Rising Yoga Therapy. Level II, a six-day intensive residential workshop, focuses on therapeutic dialogue. The first two levels are frequently combined as a 10-day training program. Level III, a six-month part-time, non-residential training, is the final and most comprehensive phase of training. It provides professional experience, knowledge, and supervision with mentors.

For Further Information

The Phoenix Rising Yoga Center is a professional training facility for Phoenix Rising Yoga Therapy Training Programs, located in West Stockbridge in the Berkshire Mountains of Massachusetts. Teacher training programs are offered there as well as at various other locations throughout the world. For further information on Phoenix Rising Yoga Therapy, including certification training, printed materials, an instructional video, books and tapes, and practitioner referrals, contact:

Phoenix Rising Yoga Center
P.O. Box 286
West Stockbridge, MA 01266
Tel: (800) 288-9642 or (413) 232-9800 (outside the United States)
Fax: (413) 232-9801
Website: *www.pryt.com*
E-mail: info@pryt.com

Suggested Further Resources

Books

Michael Lee, *Phoenix Rising Yoga Therapy: A Bridge from Body to Soul* (Health Communications, 1997). This is Michael Lee's introduction to Phoenix Rising Yoga Therapy, complete with a description of what it is, how he developed it, case histories, and exercises to try on your own.

Daniel J. Wiener, editor, *Beyond Talk Therapy: Using Movement and Expressive Techniques in Clinical Practice* (American Psychological Association, 1999). A comprehensive guide to expressive therapy techniques, this guide contains a chapter on Phoenix Rising Yoga Therapy, including case histories. To my knowledge, Michael Lee is the only yogi to be published by the American Psychological Association.

Tapes and Videos

Michael Lee has recorded some audiotapes guiding listeners through the experience of Phoenix Rising Yoga Therapy. In addition, a short informational video on Phoenix Rising Yoga Therapy is available. For further information or to order these materials, contact the Phoenix Rising Yoga Center.

Michael Lee on yoga for men:

"As a male yoga therapist using a body-mind approach, I have worked with many men over the years and continue to find that some of my deepest sessions have been with my male clients.

"The Phoenix Rising Yoga Therapy process is basically a feminine one. It is feminine insofar as it proceeds from the unknown to the known. It is nonlinear. It doesn't have a finite end or have to come to completion. It is random rather than following a set pattern. It requires more loving presence than planned action. As a result, it can sometimes get "messy." The process works from the inside out—honoring that which lies within—the dark places as well as the light.

"Now, for most men this is a strange way to work at first. Male processes usually go from the known to the unknown; are linear; get results; and follow a set and hopefully predictable pattern. And so it may seem strange, but once they get into it, men really like and appreciate the feminine process. After all, this process is not totally unknown to them. At a cellular level, it is familiar, taking them back to the womb and early infancy. It also offers men a respite from being engaged with the world—warriors ready for battle. Instead, men can now surrender to the feminine, the mystery of life, and that part of all of us that lies hidden until we are ready to engage life by letting go.

"Once men are willing to let go and engage the process, things tend to happen very quickly and easily. They embark on a journey they never could have imagined."

—Michael Lee, Founder of Phoenix Rising Therapy and Author of *Phoenix Rising Yoga Therapy—A Bridge from Body to Soul*

Chapter 10

ENDLESS YOGA

Other Traditional Approaches and Contemporary Syntheses of Yoga

The limit to man's growth is his vision; there is no end to man's self-expression. Anything which helps the reality of man to emerge from the obscure depths of his personality is yoga, whether it comes from East or West.[1]

—Sachindra Kumar Majumdar

The world of yoga is vast and seemingly endless. In addition to the many styles of yoga that have been traditionally practiced, modern-day practitioners and teachers of yoga are synthesizing the rich tools of yoga into practices that are tailor-made for special needs. This chapter summarizes some other traditional and innovative approaches to yoga in addition to those profiled in depth in the preceding chapters. You will also find information in this chapter on how you can learn more about each of these styles of yoga.

Ananda Yoga for Higher Awareness

Ananda Yoga for Higher Awareness (also known simply as Ananda Yoga) is an approach to yoga practice developed by J. Donald Walters (Swami Kriyananda), a direct disciple of Paramahansa Yogananda, author of the spiritual classic, *Autobiography of a Yogi*. Walters founded The Expanding Light Retreat (formerly the Ananda Retreat Center) in Nevada City, California, where Ananda Yoga is taught today.

Ananda Yoga is a classical style of hatha yoga that uses asanas and pranayama to awaken, experience, and control the subtle energies within oneself, especially the energies of the chakras. Its object is to use those energies to harmonize body, mind, and emotions, and, above all, to attune oneself with higher levels of awareness. Two unique features of Ananda Yoga are (1) special Energization Exercises to recharge the body with energy and (2) the practice of silent affirmations while in the poses to consciously direct the subtle energies and raise one's level of awareness. Ananda Yoga is a relatively gentle, inward experience. While not a vigorous or athletic practice, it can be challenging on the inner levels.

Ananda Yoga is offered at The Expanding Light Retreat and at Ananda teaching centers in the United States and Italy, as well as by teachers throughout the world who have been trained in this style of yoga. The Expanding Light Retreat presents an ongoing program of yoga and meditation classes, workshops, and retreats, as well as a month-long intensive residential teacher training program four times a year.

For more information on Ananda Yoga, contact:

The Expanding Light Retreat
14618 Tyler Foote Road
Nevada City, CA 95959
Tel: (800) 346-5350 or (530) 478-7518
Fax: (530) 478-7518
Website: *www.expandinglight.org* and *www.crystalclarity.com* (books and tapes)
E-mail: info@expandinglight.org

Anusara Yoga: The Heart-Centered Yoga of Flowing Grace

Anusara ("flowing with grace" in Sanskrit) Yoga is an approach to yoga developed in 1997 by American yogi John Friend, based on his many years of yoga practice. This style of yoga draws heavily on Friend's hatha yoga training in Iyengar Yoga (see Chapter 4) and his spiritual studies with Gurumayi Chidvilasananda (see "Siddha Yoga Meditation," page 105). Anusara Yoga reflects Friend's eclectic background, integrating a physically strenuous practice of hatha yoga with the spiritual focus of opening and expanding the heart center. Anusara Yoga is becoming rapidly popular throughout the United States and the rest of the world; indeed, it is one of the fastest growing hatha yoga practices in the world today, with several hundred Anusara Yoga teachers trained by Friend.

For more information on Anusara Yoga, contact:

Anusara Yoga
9400 Grogans Mill Road, Suite 200
The Woodlands, TX 77380
Tel: (888) 398-9642 or (281) 367-9763 (local and international calls)
Fax: (281) 367-2744
Website: *www.anusara.com*
E-mail: oneyoga@anusara.com

Bikram's Yoga: Yoga to the Rich and Famous

Bikram's Beginning Yoga Class (Bikram's Yoga) is an approach to yoga popularized by Bikram Choudhury, a teacher of yoga who was born in India. He first gained prominence in the 1970s when he began to offer yoga classes in Los Angeles, California. A handsome and charismatic young man who, at the age of 11, was the youngest champion in the National India Yoga Competition, Bikram quickly gained prominence in the United States as the yogi to the rich and powerful. Indeed, his roster of students includes a large number of well-known people, including entertainers such as Shirley MacLaine, athletes such as John McEnroe and Kareem Abdul-Jabbar, and a host of politicians. More recently, you may find that you more frequently see a Bikram's Yoga studio near you: Beginning in 1994, Bikram began certifying other teachers in his method. Since that time, he has trained several thousand teachers and is currently certifying 500 to 600 practitioners a year through the Yoga College of India, which he founded. His work has expanded well beyond California so that there are now more than 350 affiliated Yoga Colleges of India throughout the world.

Bikram's Yoga is based on a series of 26 yoga postures, or asanas, that are performed in a set sequence. Bikram's Yoga is typically practiced in yoga studios that are heated to a temperature of 90 to 105 degrees Fahrenheit. A typical session lasts 90 minutes. A workout in this method of yoga is thus vigorous—indeed downright sweaty—and may be of interest to men who are looking for a more strenuous approach to yoga.

The 26 postures executed systematically in Bikram's Yoga are designed to move fresh oxygen to every part of the body, helping to restore all the systems of a man's body. They can help a man to achieve proper weight, muscle tone, good health, and a sense of well-being.

For more information on Bikram's Yoga, contact:

Yoga College of India

1862 S. La Cienega

Los Angeles, CA 90035

Tel: (310) 854-5800

Fax: (310) 854-6200

Website: *www.bikramyoga.com*

E-mail: info@bikramyoga.com

Bikram's Yoga is presented in Bikram's book:

Bikram Choudhury with Bonnie Jones Reynolds, *Bikram's Beginning Yoga Class,* 2nd edition (Tarcher, 2000).

Five Tibetan Yoga: A Dynamic Yoga Flow

When we think of yoga, we often think of India. But the teachings of Hinduism and Buddhism, which first originated in India and on which traditional yoga practices are based, spread to Tibet thousands of years ago. They have influenced Tibetan thought and yoga practice for millennia. The spiritual and physical practices of Tibetan Yoga, like much knowledge about Tibet in general, remained relatively secret until recent years. Now, the secrets of Tibetan Yoga are becoming increasingly more available to Western practitioners.

The Five Tibetans are a series of five yoga exercises that are meant to be repeated in a flowing sequence for energizing body, mind, and spirit. Once mastered, each exercise in the sequence is repeated 21 times. (It is rumored that there is a "Sixth Tibetan"—sexual abstinence—but that may not be the exercise of choice for every reader!) The Five Tibetans were popularized in 1994 by a book by Christopher S. Kilham. They are based on a book written by Peter Kelder in 1939, *The Five Rites of Rejuvenation*, which presented a series of exercises taught to Kelder by a retired British army officer who claimed to have learned them from some Tibetan lamas in a Himalayan monastery. Some people believe his account is apocryphal. Whether authentically Tibetan or not, these exercises have proven very powerful for many men.

Christopher Kilham has been teaching the Five Tibetans since 1976. His book is an illustrated guide to these energizing exercises:

Christopher S. Kilham, *The Five Tibetans: Five Dynamic Exercises for Health, Energy, and Personal Power* (Inner Traditions, 1994).

There is a Website that presents an illustrated guide to the Five Tibetans. If you're interested in seeing the Five Tibetan exercises themselves, visit: *www.alchemilla.com/martial/5rites.html.*

Hidden Language of Hatha Yoga: Yoga as Self-Exploration and Reflection

Hidden Language of Hatha Yoga is a name given to the approach to yoga practiced by Swami Radha (1911–1995). Born in Germany, Swami Radha traveled to India, where she studied yoga under the guidance of Sri Swami Sivananda, one of the most seminal teachers of yoga in this century. She was the first Western woman to be initiated as a swami.

Swami Radha taught yoga throughout the world. Her approach to yoga explores the emotional, psychological, and symbolic aspects of yoga postures and practice—in what she referred to as the "hidden language" approach to yoga. Her work is preserved through the many books on yoga she authored and through the centers and organizations she established. These include the Yasodhara Ashram in Canada, the Association for the Development of Human Potential in the United States, and numerous urban teaching centers, called Radha Yoga Centers, in North America and England.

For further information on Swami Radha and her style of yoga, including a free catalog, contact:

Yasodhara Ashram Yoga Study & Retreat Centre
P.O. Box 9
Kootenay Bay, B.C. V0B 1X0
Canada
Tel: (800) 661-8711 or (250) 227-9224
Fax: (250) 227-9494
Website: *www.yasodhara.org* (for the Yasodhara Ashram in Canada) or
www.radha.org (for links to Radha Yoga Centers worldwide)
E-mail: yashram@netidea.com

For information on Swami Radha's books and tapes, and links to other pertinent sites, visit the Website of Timeless Books, the publishing arm of Yasodhara Ashram: *www.timeless.org.*

Integrative Yoga Therapy: Yoga as a Health Profession

Integrative Yoga Therapy (IYT) is an approach to yoga developed by Joseph Le Page in 1993. It offers training programs designed specifically to prepare yoga professionals to tailor yoga for use in mainstream health and wellness settings. IYT is a comprehensive and creative educational program that integrates Le Page's diverse background in yoga, educational systems and processes, world travel, and experience in healing arts.

IYT offers two training programs: A 200-hour yoga teacher training prepares individuals from a variety of backgrounds to teach therapeutic yoga classes. An advanced level yoga therapist training program is designed for yoga teachers with an interest in applying yoga therapy principles to individuals with specific health challenges.

Over the past 10 years, Le Page has trained 2,000 yoga teachers and therapists around the world. For more information on IYT, contact:

Integrative Yoga Therapy
5237 Darrow Road, #6
Hudson, OH 44236
Tel: (800) 750-9642 or (330) 655-1532
Fax: (330) 655-5892
Website: *www.iytyogatherapy.com*
E-mail: info@iytyogatherapy.com

ISHTA Yoga: The Integrated Science of Yoga

ISHTA is an acronym for the Integrated Science of Hatha, Tantra, and Ayurveda—a nomenclature coined by Alan Finger, the innovator of ISHTA Yoga. This approach to yoga was initially taught at Yoga Zone studios. Beginning in 2001, ISHTA Yoga has been taught at Be Yoga studios, located in New York City, and throughout the country by teachers trained in this style of yoga.

Alan Finger, who was born in South Africa, learned yoga from his father. He has been studying and practicing yoga for more than 40 years. His ISHTA style of practice is both physical and spiritual, and is tailored to meet each individual's need. ISHTA Yoga combines mantra recitation, kriya ("cleansing" practices), meditation, asanas, and pranayama. As appropriate, asana practice can be vigorous, with Ashtanga-style jump-backs.

For further information on ISHTA Yoga, contact:

Be Yoga
138 Fifth Avenue, 4th Floor
New York, NY 10011
Tel: (212) 647-9642
Website: *www.beyoga.com*
E-mail: info@beyoga.com

Alan Finger's approach to yoga is presented in his book:

Alan Finger and Al Bingham, *Yoga Zone Introduction to Yoga: A Beginner's Guide to Health, Fitness, and Relaxation* (Three Rivers Press, 2000).

In addition, instructional videos and tapes, as well as a link to Yoga Zone's Internet Wisdom Television station are available by visiting the Yoga Zone Website at *www.yogazone.com*.

Jivamukti Yoga: Eclectic Urban Yoga

Jivamukti (from *jivanmuktih,* "living liberated" in Sanskrit, implying one who is liberated, or enlightened, while still alive) is an eclectic synthesis of yoga practices developed by Sharon Gannon and David Life, who studied both Sivananda Yoga and Ashtanga Yoga in India. (See Chapter 5 and Chapter 6.) This style of yoga is taught and practiced at two Jivamukti Yoga Centers in New York City; one in Munich, Germany; and at other locations throughout the world by teachers who have been trained and certified by Gannon and Life. The Jivamukti Yoga Center in downtown New York City is one of the largest yoga centers in the United States. It offers more than 100 classes a week, many often filled and overflowing.

Jivamukti epitomizes hip urban style yoga. Rock celebrities and movie stars flock to its classes in the trendy Noho and fashionable Upper East Side sections of Manhattan. An issue of *Yoga Journal* included a feature article on this style of yoga with celebrity adept practitioner Sting on its cover.

Jivamukti Yoga is noted for the physically challenging rigor of its asana practice, as well as by its psychological and spiritual depth. Jivamukti's emphasis on ethical vegetarianism helps to awaken in the practitioner a need to protect the earth, the environment, and all the animals and plants that share the planet with us.

Each class is one hour and 35 minutes long and integrates chanting, breathing exercises, music, meditation, and ancient, traditional sacred scriptures into a vigorous physical practice that includes a vinyasa flowing sequence of asanas (see "Vinyasa Yoga," page 108). It provides a blueprint for incorporating the physical and spiritual aspects of yoga into modern man's life.

For further information on Jivamukti Yoga, contact:

Jivamukti Yoga Center

404 Lafayette Street, 3rd Floor

New York, NY 10003

Tel: (800) 295-6814 or (212) 353-0214

Fax: (212) 995-1313

Website: *www.jivamuktiyoga.com*

E-mail: info@jivamuktiyoga.com

The principles of Jivamukti Yoga are presented in the following book:

Sharon Gannon and David Life, *Jivamukti Yoga: Practices for Liberating Body and Soul* (Ballantine, 2002). Also available by Gannon and Life: *The Art of Yoga* (Stewart, Tabori, and Chang, 2002).

Self-Realization Fellowship: Paramahansa Yogananda's Legacy

Paramahansa Yogananda (1893–1952) was one of the most famous yogis of the 20th century. In 1920, he was sent from India to the United States by his guru with the encouraging message: "You are the one I have chosen to spread the message of *Kriya Yoga* in the West.... The scientific technique of God-realization will ultimately spread in all lands, and aid in harmonizing the nations through man's personal, transcendental perception of the Infinite Father."[2] Yogananda initiated thousands of individuals into the practice of Kriya Yoga, a special technique for stilling the mind and withdrawing the energy from sensory perceptions in order to ultimately attain personal experience of God. His *Autobiography of a Yogi* has become a classic around the world. Yogananda's teachings emphasized the spiritual role of yoga on the path to self-realization. His work is carried on today by Self-Realization Fellowship, the nonprofit organization that he founded in 1920 for that purpose. The Self-Realization Fellowship offers guided retreats, classes, and lectures on the teachings of Paramahansa Yogananda; a series of home-study lessons; and it sponsors events at affiliated branches and centers around the world.

For further information on the teachings and legacy of Paramahansa Yogananda, contact:

Self-Realization Fellowship

3880 San Rafael Avenue, Dept. 9W

Los Angeles, CA 90065-3298

Tel: (323) 225-2471 (9 a.m. to 5 p.m. Pacific Time)

Fax: (323) 225-5088

Website: *www.yogananda.org*

The following book written by Paramahansa Yogananda and first published in 1946 remains a perennial classic of yoga:

Paramahansa Yogananda, *Autobiography of a Yogi,* 13th edition (Self-Realization Fellowship, 1998).

Siddha Yoga Meditation: The Grace of the Master

Siddha Yoga meditation is an approach to yoga bequeathed by Swami Muktananda (1908–1982), a noted teacher in India and disciple of Bhagawan Nityananda of Ganeshpuri, regarded as one of the great saints of modern India. *Siddha* literally means "a perfect human being" in Sanskrit. Siddha Yoga meditation uses a variety of techniques, such as chanting, meditation, selfless service, and mantra repetition, as ways to attain enlightenment and perfection.

The most complete reference about the Siddha Yoga path is Swami Muktananda's spiritual autobiography, *Play of Consciousness*. Siddha Yoga meditation is one of the most widely practiced spiritual approaches today. Gurumayi Chidvilasananda, Swami Muktananda's chosen successor and the current master of the tradition, continues to guide Siddha Yoga students today. Siddha Yoga meditation is currently practiced in a few ashrams and hundreds of centers around the world.

For more information on Siddha Yoga meditation, contact its international head-quarters at:

SYDA Foundation
371 Brickman Road
South Fallsburg, NY 12779
Tel: (845) 434-2000
Website: *www.siddhayoga.org*
E-mail: Info@siddhayoga.org

The following book is the classic text on Swami Muktananda and his teachings:
Swami Muktananda, *Play of Consciousness: A Spiritual Autobiography* (SYDA Foundation, 2000).

The following books are helpful to newcomers of this path:
Gurumayi Chidvilasananda, *Inner Treasures* (SYDA Foundation, 1995).
Swami Muktananda, *Where Are You Going?* (SYDA Foundation, 1989).

Thai Yoga Massage

Thai Yoga Massage is an approach to bodywork that combines yoga with focused touch. Tracing its origins to the temples and martial arts traditions of Thailand, Thai Yoga Massage is practiced in pairs. One partner assists another in yoga postures while applying pressure with the hands along lines and special points of energy in the body.

One of the world's foremost teachers and practitioners of Thai Yoga Massage is Kam Thye Chow, who presents the principles of this healing therapy in his illustrated instructional guidebook:

Kam Thye Chow, *Thai Yoga Massage: A Dynamic Therapy for Physical Well-Being and Spiritual Energy* (Healing Arts, 2002).

TriYoga: Energetic, Dance-like Yoga

Kali Ray TriYoga, founded by Kali Ray, an American yogini, is a systematic method to yoga that includes the full spectrum of traditional practices. TriYoga's hatha yoga method, TriYoga Flows, is the union of postures, breath, and focus. By the nature of its origin, this threefold practice is deeply meditative, promoting relaxation and inner peace. TriYoga is a particularly flowing style of yoga, with levels ranging from basic to advanced. It incorporates wave-like spinal movements that can help men build strength, flexibility, and endurance, while uniting body and mind. TriYoga teachers offer this style of yoga in a wide variety of settings that include such mainstream venues as Duke University, hospitals and clinics, the United States Senate, and even corporate giants such as Intel and Hewlett-Packard.

For further information on TriYoga, contact:

Kali Ray TriYoga International HQ
P.O. Box 6367

Malibu, CA 90264
Tel: (310) 589-0600
Fax: (310) 589-0783
Website: *www.triyoga.com*
E-mail: info@triyoga.com

Urban Yoga: Yoga Joins the Gym Workout

Urban Yoga is an approach to yoga that you may see offered in a class setting by your local gym or yoga studio. This nomenclature for a style of yoga first started to appear around the beginning of the 1980s, and has become even more widespread since then. While there is not necessarily one particular style of Urban Yoga, in general Urban Yoga refers to an eclectic blend of traditional hatha yoga postures combined with other activities that you may find offered in a gym setting. This may include aerobics choreographed to music in a high-energy spin-off. Another style may incorporate yoga practices with body-strengthening exercises. A more relaxing approach may emphasize breathing techniques, stretching exercises, and restorative poses to complement a more traditional weightlifting workout. Whatever the ingredients, Urban Yoga can appeal to men who want to de-stress by combining the traditional benefits of hatha yoga with a gym-environment workout. If you see a class in Urban Yoga advertised near you, check out what the ingredients of that particular class are. Urban Yoga may be just the right thing for you—whether you live in a city or the countryside.

Viniyoga: Yoga Tailored to the Individual

Viniyoga is an approach to yoga popularized by American yogi Gary Kraftsow. It is not so much the name of a yoga as an approach to developing a personal practice of yoga. Kraftsow began his studies of yoga with the highly respected East Indian teacher, T.K.V. Desikachar, son of Sri Krishnamacharya, one of the 20th century's greatest yoga masters. With Desikachar's blessing, Kraftsow established the American Viniyoga Institute (AVI), where he and his wife, Mirka, make the teachings of Viniyoga accessible to the public.

Viniyoga is characterized by its emphasis on the breath and the flowing manner in which postures are executed. It incorporates meditation, prayer, and ritual. Viniyoga draws upon the teachings of the South Indian yogi and sage Nathamuni (circa 800 C.E.) Nathamuni traces his lineage to Patanjali (believed to have lived between 200 and 500 C.E.), who, as the author of the oldest text on yoga, is sometimes referred to as the "father of yoga." Nathamuni taught that as we grow, the methods we use must be modified and the very purpose of our practice changed.

Viniyoga is thus ideally suited to the man (or boy) who wants to tailor a yoga practice suited to his individual needs—in particular, in respect to his age. For children, Viniyoga practice supports the balanced growth and development of the body and mind. For adult men, the practice aims to safeguard health and promote the ability to be productive in the world. For senior men, Viniyoga practice helps to maintain health while inspiring a deeper quest for self-realization. (For more guidance on how yoga can help men at different stages of their life's journey, see Chapter 11, which reflects much of the teachings of Viniyoga.)

For further information on Viniyoga, contact:

American Viniyoga Institute, LLC

P.O. Box 88

Makawao, HI 96768

Tel: (808) 572-1414

Fax: (808) 573-2000 or (800) 572-5775

Website: *www.viniyoga.com*

E-mail: info@viniyoga.com

Gary Kraftsow has published two books that explore his approach to yoga:

Gary Kraftsow, *Yoga for Wellness: Healing with the Timeless Teachings of Viniyoga* (Penguin, 1999). With more than 1,000 illustrations, this is Gary Kraftsow's introduction to his complete system of Viniyoga. It presents case studies and specific yoga sequences for individual needs.

————, *Yoga for Transformation: Ancient Teachings and Practices for Healing the Body, Mind, and Heart* (Penguin, 2002). In his second book, Gary Kraftsow makes the inner teachings of yoga accessible, presenting techniques that treat not only the physical body, but also the emotions and mind for transformation at the level of the heart and soul.

Vinyasa Yoga: The Yoga of Flowing, Connected Movement

Vinyasa Yoga is a style of yoga that can represent a variety of yoga practices. *Vinyasa* literally means "uninterrupted flow" in Sanskrit. What typically characterizes styles of yoga that call themselves Vinyasa is the flowing way in which the sequence of postures is connected. In a Vinyasa Yoga class, each movement is often performed in a flowing sequence, without stopping and starting, with each movement executed in synch with the breath.

A number of styles of yoga incorporate this sense of connection and flow—such as Ashtanga Yoga, Jivamukti Yoga, and White Lotus Yoga. If you should see a class advertised as Vinyasa Yoga, check with the instructor to find out more about it so that you can understand better what the instructor has in mind regarding "uninterrupted flow"—some Vinyasa Yoga classes can be quite strenuous while others can be more relaxing and restorative.

White Lotus Yoga: Flowing Power Yoga

White Lotus Yoga is a synthesis of the major styles and traditions of yoga and the expression of many years of teaching by Tracey Rich and Ganga White, who have studied and taught yoga extensively around the world for more than 36 years. White Lotus Yoga combines the precision of Iyengar Yoga (see Chapter 4), the wisdom of classical yoga, and the flowing sequences and special breathing practices of both Ashtanga Yoga (see Chapter 6) and Vinyasa Yoga with White's own experience with thousands of students. The approach emphasizes cycling one's practice by alternating different styles of yoga, tuning one's yoga practice to one's own needs, and is taught in a non-dogmatic, open-minded manner.

White Lotus Yoga is taught and practiced at the White Lotus Foundation, a residential mountain retreat center overlooking Santa Barbara, California. Teacher training and certification is offered in 16-day intensive residential retreats that cover asana practice, pranayama, yoga philosophy, teacher training, professional issues, and a variety of other topics. Other offerings include a variety of workshops and programs such as three- to four-day retreats and a week of White Lotus Yoga.

For further information on White Lotus Yoga, contact:

White Lotus Yoga Foundation

2500 San Marcos Pass

Santa Barbara, CA 93105

Tel: (805) 964-1944 or (800) 544-3569 (product orders only)

Fax: (805) 964-9617

Website: *www.whitelotus.org*

E-mail: info@whitelotus.org

Ganga White's partner approach to yoga is presented in his book:

Ganga White, *Double Yoga: A New System for Total Body Health* (White Lotus Foundation, 1998). This book, as well as a series of videos, is available by contacting White Lotus Yoga.

Yogaerobics: Aerobicizing With Yoga

Similar to Urban Yoga, Yogaerobics is a generic term for a class that you might see offered at your local gym or in a yoga or exercise studio near you. Generally, it refers to an eclectic blend of hatha yoga and traditional aerobics. Should you come across a Yogaerobics class in your area and be interested in it, check with the instructor to see exactly what the class entails.

Yogassage: Yoga for Two

Yogassage is a recently coined term that combines the notions of yoga and massage. Yogassage is often used to refer to yoga that is practiced with a partner. Practicing yoga with a partner—whether a loved one or a workout mate—can be a lot of fun. In addition, you can get an even better stretch and other enhanced benefits when someone helps you go more deeply into a yoga posture. For this reason, there is a separate chapter in *Yoga for Men* titled "Partnered Yoga" (Chapter 15) devoted to this subject—complete with illustrated instructions on representative partnered yoga exercises.

Nateshvar Ken Scott is one yoga innovator who has developed an approach to yoga that he calls "Yogassage." It is similar to Thai massage. One partner completely relaxes and receives, while the other gives. Yogassage incorporates yoga stretches with the creative use of hands, arms, elbows, knees, and feet in an especially nurturing and opening practice. For further information, contact Nateshvar Ken Scott by telephone or via the Internet at:

Nateshvar Ken Scott

Telephone: (250) 358-2880

Website: *www.nateshvar.com*

E-mail: kamini@netidea.com

Yogilates: Yoga Joins Pilates

Yogilates represents a marriage of yoga with a system of wellness and fitness known as the Pilates Method. The Pilates Method is a series of movement exercises developed by German-born Joseph Pilates (1880–1967) in the 1920s. These exercises are designed to make people more aware of their bodies while stretching and strengthening muscles, opening joints, and releasing tension. Interest in the Pilates Method has grown enormously in recent years. The exercises that form part of this method are a natural complement to yoga postures. Teachers who are trained in both the Pilates Method and yoga are now incorporating the two practices together in a system known as Yogilates.

Jonathon Urla is a well-known practitioner and an author on Yogilates. You can find out more information about Yogilates by contacting him at:

Yogilates

309 East 87th Street, #6G

New York, NY 10128

Tel: (877) 964-4528

Website: *www.yogilates.com*

E-mail: info@yogilates.com

The principles of Yogilates are presented in his book:

Jonathon Urla, *Yogilates: Integrating Yoga and Pilates for Complete Fitness, Strength, and Flexibility* (HarperInformation, 2002).

Mark Donato on yoga for men:

"In my observation, men are more externally oriented and controlling of their environment than women are. The problem is that when they are busy working their butts off to support their family (or themselves), they lose touch with their personal environment—i.e., their body and breath. Even men who are physically fit and work out a lot, oftentimes have little awareness of their bodies when they get into yoga class. ('Breath? What's that?' they may ask.)

"One of the biggest challenges men in general have in yoga class is their release of control. Just allowing themselves to sit and watch the breath. To watch the mind as we watch the breath, and accept what comes up. Yoga is about taking an honest look at ourselves; and we may not always like what we see. That's why lifting weights and working on the machines at gyms is much easier. Because we can just pummel through our workouts without any sense of mindfulness.

"Another reason yoga is beneficial for men is prostate health: cobbler pose, eagle pose, root lock, for instance, are good for promoting prostate health."

—Mark Donato, Teacher of his own signature approach to yoga, Core Yoga, at
Om Yoga Center, New York City

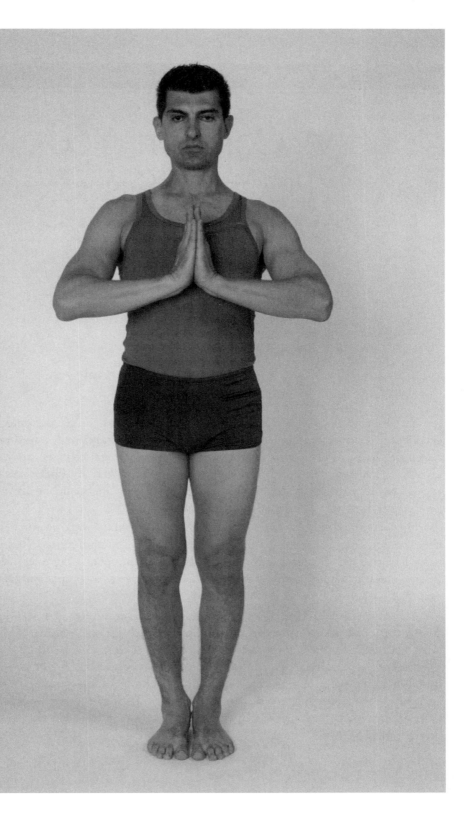

A Complete Yoga
Practice Session
for Men

The best way to begin the practice of yoga is to learn under the guidance of a good, experienced teacher. Nothing can compare with the individualized, hands-on training such a teacher can provide. With the growing popularity of yoga, chances are that you can find a yoga studio, center, class, or teacher located close to you. By understanding the various approaches to yoga presented in *Yoga for Men*, you'll be able to make an informed, intelligent selection of one that's just right for you.

However, you may be eager to learn about some basic yoga postures if you're new to yoga, or you may be interested in deepening your understanding of certain common postures if you're already practicing yoga. This section presents a complete, illustrated, step-by-step guide to a yoga session for men, which can serve as a companion guide to your yoga practice.

According to yoga lore, Shiva, the great yoga master, created 8.4 million asanas. Fortunately, you don't need to practice all of those asanas to get the benefits of yoga! In practice, most teachers of yoga incorporate anywhere from several to a hundred or so postures in their overall repertoire. A typical 60- to 90-minute yoga class might contain one to two dozen different asanas that are carefully sequenced to provide a complete workout for body and mind. Some teachers even claim that certain powerful poses—such as Downward-Facing Dog, which is presented in the Sun Salutation series—can give you nearly all the benefits of yoga.

The following yoga postures were carefully selected to guide you through a basic, Complete Yoga Session that you should be able to complete in an hour or less. This practice session includes one flowing series of poses followed by a dozen or so yoga asanas that will help you become more flexible, gain strength, and improve circulation and joint mobility. This session has been designed to help you restore and energize not only your body, but also your mind and spirit. The poses in this yoga program are those that you will find included most regularly in hatha yoga classes, no matter what the particular style or approach to performing the exercise postures is. They are the basic postures for healthy, stress-free living.

While the physical asanas of yoga help to stretch, relax, and restore, they can also be physically challenging. You should only practice the poses in this yoga practice session if you are in good physical condition. If you have any physical problems, particularly in the areas of the neck, back, shoulders, or knees, as well as any circulatory or other health problems, you should consult with your physician before trying the poses. Whenever you practice yoga, pay close attention to your body and only perform postures within your level of comfort. The poses in this yoga practice session are presented for informational purposes only, not for medical or therapeutic treatment. They cannot fully teach the techniques described, but rather offer suggestions for yoga practice that should be integrated with instruction and supervision from competent teachers. If you have any particular health or other concerns, always check with your doctor to get his or her approval before embarking upon any exercise program.

Before you begin "A Complete Yoga Practice Session for Men," read through the in-structions for the practice from beginning to end to familiarize yourself with the program. Then, when you feel ready, begin your own personal practice of yoga. To help you get started, you might try reading the instructions for each pose into a tape recorder and play them back as you follow along with them. Even better, you might try doing this yoga session with a friend or family member who can read you the instructions as you embark upon, or deepen, your yoga practice journey.

The postures in the session that follow are accompanied by illustrations of various yoga teachers and students demonstrating the positions. These models represent diverse age groups and body types, as well as varying levels of proficiency in yoga. They are all united in the common goal of wanting to share their enthusiasm for yoga with you. As are most of the readers of this book, they are real men doing real yoga.

As you do your yoga practice, be kind to yourself. Remember: There is no "perfect" way to do each pose. There is only your way. Respect your limits. Always bear in mind that yoga is not a competitive sport. You don't need to feel that you *have* to compete with anyone—including yourself—when you do yoga. Regard your yoga practice as an opportunity to become more mindful and better aware of yourself and your limitations. Allow your yoga practice to be an opportunity for increasing your level of self-acceptance. Be aware of areas of holding, of poses that seem more difficult to perform, as well as any other awareness that comes to you. In this way, you'll learn to know your body better, and, with regular practice, help to optimize its functioning.

And last, but not least, remember that yoga can be fun! So have fun as you start out on your own personal practice of yoga.

The Basic Postures for Healthy, Stress-Free Living: Preparing for Your Yoga Practice Session

In preparation for your yoga practice, find a place where you will be able to practice comfortably. You will need an uncluttered space where you will be able to stretch out and move about freely. If necessary, move any furniture or other objects that might intrude on your practice out of the way. You will be working on a smooth, flat, nonskid surface on the floor. Ideally, a bare wooden floor on which you can place a yoga "sticky mat" to help enhance balance and prevent skidding is best. (See Chapter 17 to find out more about yoga props and how you can obtain them.) For seated postures and those performed when lying on the floor, some type of cushioning—a pillow, bolster, folded sticky mat, blanket, or towel—will help to provide support and make your practice more comfortable. You will probably find it easier to perform standing poses by standing directly on a yoga mat or a bare wood floor rather than on a carpeted surface. This will give you a firmer footing for added balance and stability.

Wear loose, comfortable clothing. A T-shirt and shorts might be just the ideal attire. It is best if you are barefoot while you perform your yoga session, as this will enable your feet to have the most secure contact with the floor in standing positions. If you would like to experiment with using props, you can have accessories ready to help you. These could include a yoga belt or rope to help you in some of the stretching poses and a small wooden or foam block, or a strong and sturdy straight-backed chair or table to help support you in some of the balancing poses. You may also find it handy to have a blanket nearby to place over yourself in the final relaxation pose, as you may find that your body feels cooler when you assume the final resting pose at the end of this yoga session.

Surya Namaskara: Sun Salutation

Many yoga classes begin with the execution of a yoga exercise called *Surya Namaskara* (literally "Salute to the Sun" or "Sun Salutation"). This is not technically an asana, but rather a series of flowing movements that incorporate a number of different postures into one exercise. The Sun Salutation presented here synthesizes the elements of many widely practiced approaches to yoga. It is designed to warm up the body for the postures that will follow during the Complete Yoga Session. The Sun Salutation is composed of a number of movements performed in sequence. These movements flow into each other and help to stretch the body and improve the circulation of blood so that your yoga practice will be even more beneficial. As you perform each sequence of the Sun Salutation series in succession, pay attention to your breath. Perform each movement as indicated in the instructions with an inhalation or an exhalation. As you practice yoga, let your breath be your friend and guide.

Opening Stance: Tadasana—Mountain Pose

To begin the Sun Salutation series, stand at the front and center of your mat if you have one. Otherwise, just stand on the floor with the inside of your big toes and heels touching. Take a moment to feel that your toes are planted firmly on the floor and that you are balanced evenly on the inside and outside surface edges of your feet. Your weight should

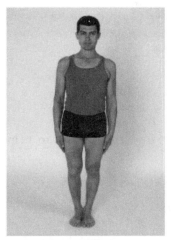

Fig. YPS.1a: Mountain Pose

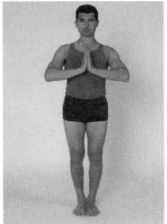

Fig. YPS.1b: Hands at Center Breast

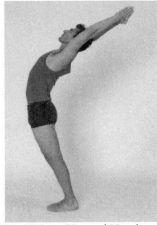

Fig. YPS.1c: Upward Hands Pose (Arms Alongside Ears)

also be evenly distributed among the back, middle, and front of the bottom surfaces of your feet. Allow your thighs to be firm and engaged, your tailbone pointing toward the floor. Allow your chest to be open and expansive, sternum facing forward and up. Allow your head to be perpendicular to the floor, your eyes are open, and your gaze is soft and neutral, focused at a spot on the wall directly in front of you. Allow your arms to hang by your sides, palms and inside surface of the fingers facing toward and touching the outside of your thighs. Check again to be sure your weight is evenly distributed on your feet. Contract your thighs, as you remain active even while standing still.

This is *tadasana*, or "Mountain Pose." Imagine yourself as a mountain, feet securely grounded in the earth, your body rising, fully supported, just like a mountain. Take a few full breaths as you acknowledge how your body feels in this position. See if you can make your weight even more firmly balanced over your feet.

Position 1: Namaskar—Hands at Center Breast

Exhale as you gently place your hands, palms touching, in front of your chest, in a position known as *namaskar*. The placement of the hands with the palms touching is sometimes popularly referred to as *namaste*, or "Prayer Position." It is named this because it calls to mind the position of the hands during prayer in many cultures and traditions, but it has absolutely nothing to do with religion in the context of yoga practice. You are placing your hands here in this way in order to center yourself and prepare for the sequence of movements that follow. In addition, you are practicing a *mudra*, or yogic "seal" with your hands, sealing in the circuit of energy throughout your entire body, and showing your respect and attentiveness to the practice that is to follow. Take a few moments to take a few full, deep, clearing, energizing breaths as you center yourself for the movements to follow in surya namaskara.

Position 2: Urdhva Hastasana— Upward Hands Pose (Arms Alongside Ears)

Inhale as you gradually move your hands out to your sides and up over your head until your arms are straight alongside your ears. Allow the palms of your hands to meet above your head, as in Prayer Position. Look up toward your fingertips as you gently arch backward. This position is known as *urdhva hastasana* in Sanskrit (see Fig. YPS.1c).

Position 3: Uttanasana— Standing Forward Bend

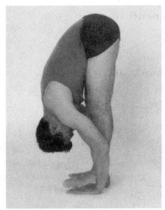

Exhale as you dive forward, arms out to the sides, as though you are executing a swan dive. Keep your lower back and torso as straight and erect as possible, then fold forward, belly over the thighs. Try not to round forward as you allow your head to move toward the floor. Place your palms on the floor, parallel to and outside of your feet, fingertips in line with the toes. See if you can touch your knees with your head. If you are able, allow your legs to remain straight. If the palms of your hands do not reach the floor with straight legs, bend your knees until your palms are firmly on the floor. If that is too challenging for you, then simply let your hands reach as close to the ground as possible. Be patient with your-

Fig. YPS.1d: Standing Forward Bend

self: With regular practice, you will gain greater flexibility and will be able to stretch further and deeper in this position. This posture is known as *uttanasana*. It literally means "Intense Stretch," but is commonly referred to as "Standing Forward Bend."

Position 4: Flat Back Pose

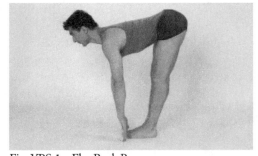

Retain your breath for a moment in Standing Forward Bend as you allow your back to rise to a flat, straight position, as perpendicular to the floor as possible. Your fingertips are still in line with the toes, but your palms lift up off the floor to help you straighten and widen your back, especially the upper back and shoulder areas. Look up.

Fig. YPS.1e: Flat Back Pose

For some readers who already practice yoga, this may be a new variation on the Sun Salutation series that you customarily perform. This flat back pose forms part of the series of movements that are performed in Ashtanga Yoga. It is included here because of the beneficial effect it has on opening the back and shoulders.

Position 5: Lunge Pose—Right Leg Back

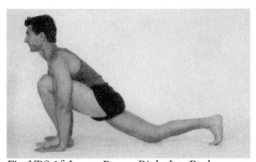

Inhale as you step your right leg back and extend it behind you so that your right knee is on the floor. Your left foot is positioned between

Fig. YPS.1f: Lunge Pose—Right Leg Back

your two hands. It stays bent and forms a right angle to the floor with your left lower leg. Your right leg is in a lunge position in a strong stretch. As you breathe, press more deeply into your right hip to increase the benefits of the stretch.

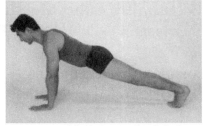

Fig. YPS.1g: Plank Pose—Modified Push-up Position

Position 6: Plank Pose—Modified Push-up Position

Retain your breath as you lift up your left foot and leg and bring them back to form a parallel line with your right leg and foot. Your two legs and feet are together, lifted in a straight line off the floor in a modified push-up position. You are now in a position popularly referred to as "Plank Pose." Your hands are under your shoulders, palms on the floor, fingers pointing straight out in front of you. Your arms are straight, with the insides of the elbows and forearms facing forward. Your torso is parallel to the floor. Contract your abdomen to maintain your straight, active position—your entire body forms a line as straight as a plank from head to toe.

Position 7: Ahstang Pranam—Knees, Chest, and Chin to the Floor

Exhale as you slowly, and with control, lower yourself down so that your knees, chest, and chin touch the floor. Your pelvis and the mid-section of your torso remain lifted off the floor. Your feet are flexed and touching the floor, toes curled under. Your hands are placed with palms flat on the floor next to your shoulders. Your elbows are raised and your upper arms are aligned to be as straight, close, and parallel to your torso as possible. This position is known as *ashtang pranam*—"Eight-

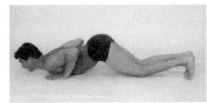

Fig. YPS.1h: Knees, Chest, and Chin to the Floor

Limbed Prostration"—because only eight "limbs" of your body are in contact with the floor (your feet, knees, hands, chest, and chin). The name of this pose reminds us that in this series of movements that comprise the Sun Salutation, we are prostrating ourselves before the sun.

Position 8: Bhujangasana— Cobra Pose

Inhale as you gradually slide your chin, neck, and head forward—up and off the floor—as you maintain your hand placement securely on the floor. Allow your belly and lower torso to sink onto the floor as your upper back arches up from the floor. Point your toes so that the top surface of each foot rests in contact with the floor. Your arms straighten as you lift up into what

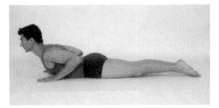

Fig. YPS.1i: Cobra Pose

is known as *bhujangasana*, or "Cobra Pose." This posture provides a strong backward bend, so lift your chest, pull down and away with your shoulders, and arch your upper back as much as you can to get the greatest stretch possible.

Position 9: Adho Mukha Svanasana—Downward-Facing Dog

Exhale as you curl your toes under and lift your buttocks up into the air so that your body forms an inverted V in relation to the floor. Allow your feet to rotate back completely so that your toes are flexed and you are supported on the balls of your toes. Allow your head to hang between

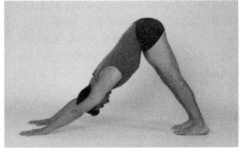
Fig. YPS.1j: Downward-Facing Dog

your elbows, your gaze directed up and back toward your navel. Draw your sit-bones up into the air. Lift your shoulders out and away from the ears. Continue to broaden your shoulders and upper back. Keep your legs as straight as possible. Your feet should be hip-width distance (4 to 6 inches) apart, your heels pressing toward the floor. If possible, keep your feet, heels included, flat on the floor. If this is challenging for you, it's alright to let your heels lift up off the floor while the balls of your feet stay firmly planted on the ground. If the pose is still challenging you, bend your knees as much as necessary. Hold this position for five deep breaths. This position is known as *adho mukha svanasana*, or "Downward-Facing Dog." You are giving a wonderful stretch and massage to your entire body—back, arms, shoulders, pelvis, and legs. In fact, some yogis maintain that this pose alone benefits virtually every part of your body. Take several full, deep, relaxed breaths in Downward-Facing Dog.

Position 10: Lunge Pose—Left Leg Back

Inhale as you simultaneously lower your torso and lift and step your right foot forward, placing it between your two hands. If necessary, use your hands to help bring the right foot forward. Allow your left knee to touch the floor as you enter into a lunge position . Your right knee is between your two hands. Breathe deeply as you press into your left hip.

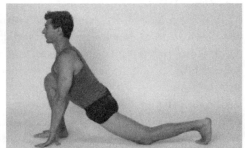
Fig. YPS.1k: Lunge Pose—Left Leg Back

Position 11: Uttanasana—Standing Forward Bend

Exhale as you lift your left leg, bringing it forward so that your left foot is parallel to and touches your right foot. Your hands are on the floor outside of your feet, fingertips in line with the toes, at the front center of your yoga mat or space. Keep your legs as straight as possible and allow the head

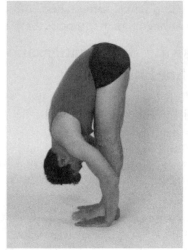
Fig. YPS.1l: Standing Forward Bend

to hang as low and close to the floor as possible. Try not to lock your knees. To help keep your legs as straight as possible, try contracting your quadriceps. To help you stretch further forward, try folding your torso at the hips—as though there is a hinge at your hips that allows you to press and fold your upper body forward. This will help you keep your back as straight as possible rather than rounding forward. You are now, once again, in uttanasana, or Standing Forward Bend.

Position 12: Urdhva Hastasana—Upward Hands Pose (Arms Alongside Ears)

Inhale as you raise your arms out to the sides and execute a reverse swan dive. Bring the palms of your hands together to touch above your head. Try to keep the arms straight with the inside of your upper arms, parallel to and alongside your ears. Bend back as far as you can. Check to make sure that you are not dropping your neck back. Rather, keep your head and neck in line with your arms to avoid any excessive stretch.

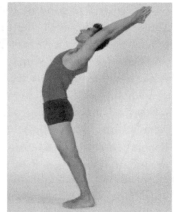

Fig. YPS.1m: Upward Hands Pose—Arms Alongside Ears

Position 13: Namaskar—Hands at Center Breast

Exhale as you allow your arms to float down and your torso to return to a straight vertical line. Bring your palms together in front of your chest in Prayer Position.

Closing Stance: Tadasana— Mountain Pose

Complete this portion of the Sun Salutation by bringing your hands down alongside your body to assume the position of Mountain Pose, which formed the Opening Stance to the Sun Salutation. Breathe several deep breaths to center yourself and integrate the benefits of the Sun Salutation. Take a moment to see how you feel after practicing the first portion of one round of the Sun Salutation series.

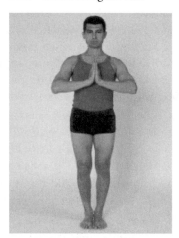

Fig. YPS.1n: Hands at Center Breast

Completing Surya Namaskara: Sun Salutation

To complete your Salute to the Sun, repeat the preceding movements, reversing the order of your lunges: Step the left leg back (Position 5) and forward (Position 10), instead of the right. Performing these two movement sequences constitutes one full round of Sun Salutation.

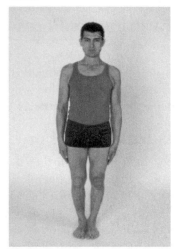

Fig. YPS.1o: Mountain Pose

Once you've done the Sun Salutation on both sides of the body, congratulate yourself! You've just completed one full round of the Sun Salutation series. If this is your first time practicing yoga, you've just taken one of the most important steps that you can in your practice of yoga and your pursuit of healthy, stress-free living. If you're already practicing yoga, you already know the many benefits of the Sun Salutation.

This one sequence of movements provides a nearly perfect full-body workout. When performed correctly and completely, it stretches, tones, and strengthens virtually every muscle group in the body. It also helps to improve circulation and improve joint mobility. It is both relaxing and energizing at the same time. No wonder the ancient sages used this practice to start their days and salute the sun—the symbol of the divine radiance within each one of us. If you don't have time to do a full yoga routine, doing just several rounds of Sun Salutation during the day can be an important ingredient in your overall fitness and well-being program.

If you have been practicing yoga for some time, you might want to vary your practice of the Sun Salutation series by incorporating a greater sense of flow into your routine. This will help you experience a more flowing, rather than static, approach to yoga practice. If you'd like to challenge yourself further in Sun Salutation series, execute several rounds of Sun Salutation without stopping, flowing steadily and rhythmically on each inhalation and exhalation from one position to the next. In this way, you'll be incorporating *vinyasa*, or uninterrupted seamless flow, with the breath into your practice.

As you practice yoga, learn to listen to your body. Be sure not to push yourself beyond your limits. Be aware of your body's needs, which can change from day to day and from pose to pose. Yoga can be challenging, but it is not meant to be stressful. If you need to, lighten up on your practice and modify the poses to suit your individual needs. Yoga can be both invigorating and restorative. Remember to tune in to and pay attention to your breath: Your breath is your greatest teacher.

If you are new to yoga, or are still working to develop your flexibility and stamina while performing yoga, it's important to be able to rest and renew yourself during your yoga practice. The following asanas are powerful restorative poses.

Restorative Poses

All of the poses in this Complete Yoga Session are optional. If you feel as though you'd like to skip one or more of the postures, feel free to do so, or rest in between or in place of any of the postures. The following asanas are yoga postures that are ideal for resting between more active postures or whenever you feel that you need a bit of time for yourself.

Balasana: Boy's or Child's Pose

Balasana, which literally means "Boy's Pose," is most commonly referred to as "Child's Pose." It provides a gentle stretch to the back, shoulders, legs, and feet while allowing you to rest in a place of calm and peace. It's a posture that you can assume whenever you need to rest and relax—not only during your yoga practice session, but also at any time during a stressful day when you may need a bit of time for yourself. Following are step-by-step instructions for entering into Child's Pose.

Come to a kneeling position on the floor. You can either keep your legs close together or let your knees and upper legs spread out to the side as the big toes of your feet come together behind you, the top surfaces of the feet in contact with the floor. As you exhale, allow your upper body to fold down over your thighs, forehead resting on the floor. If you can, let your buttocks rest securely on the heels of your feet. If not, let your buttocks rest gently raised off your heels, yet as low to the ground as possible. Stretch your arms out in front of you. To achieve a long, full stretch for your back and shoulder area, walk your fingertips forward until you feel a stretch along your entire back—from the base of your neck, across your upper and middle back, all the way down to your tailbone. Rest like a little boy.

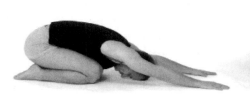

Fig. YPS.2a: Child's Pose With Arms Stretched in Front

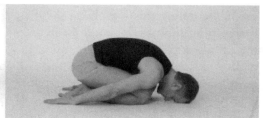

Fig. YPS.2b: Child's Pose With Arms Along Sides of the Body

As a variation of Child's Pose, you can also try bringing your arms down alongside your torso, palms facing up (see Fig. YPS. 2b). The placement of your arms and hands may help to relax the shoulders and back. Feel the area of your lower back widening and expanding in this variation of Child's Pose. Feel the area of your upper back and shoulders widening simultaneously. See if you can rest your buttocks even closer to or on your heels in this variation—you may find a pleasant deepening of the release and stretch in your lower back as you do so.

As an additional variation, you can experiment with making a "pillow" out of your hands to support your neck and head. Place your hands one on top of the other, palms facing down, under your forehead. Keep your buttocks positioned toward your heels while you allow your neck and head to relax.

Stay in any variation of Boy's or Child's Pose you choose for as long as you feel you need to. Breathe slowly, deeply, fully and rhythmically. Allow the breath to circulate throughout your entire body. Feel yourself relaxing and releasing even further into the posture with each breath. Holding this position for half a minute to several minutes can be deeply calming and restorative.

Savasana: Corpse Pose

Savasana literally means "Corpse Pose" or "Dead Man's Pose." It is a posture of complete relaxation and abandon. While this asana is frequently assumed at the end of a yoga practice session, you can also use it to rest between yoga poses. In some hatha yoga traditions, savasana is used as a transition between more active yoga poses in order to allow the body to assimilate and integrate the benefits of one pose before continuing on to another. Try savasana for yourself to see how it can help to calm your mind and reduce tension and anxiety.

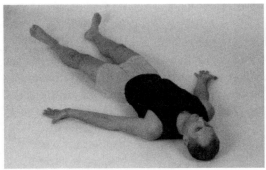

Fig. YPS.3: Corpse Pose

Lie down easefully on your back on a comfortable, padded surface. Allow your legs to spread evenly out to your sides several inches or more away from the midline of your body. Try to ensure that the feet are evenly turned out. They should ideally be in a neutral position—neither flexed nor extended—and relaxed. Allow your arms to rest alongside your torso, angled out slightly, backs of the arms in contact with the floor and palms facing up. The back of your head should be resting comfortably on the floor. Check to make sure that your neck is not arched backward or forward. It should be in an even, neutral position so that your face is parallel to the ceiling and your nose is pointing in a straight line directly toward the ceiling. If you need to, place a pillow, folded towel, or blanket under the back of your head to rest it in a more comfortable position. Also, check to make sure that your shoulder blades are relaxed. They should be wide and in contact with the floor. Allow the sacrum to rest on the floor and the lumbar spine to retain its natural curve. You may find it more comfortable to place pillows, folded towels, or a blanket under your knees: This helps to relieve any pressure on the lower back so that it can release even further toward the floor.

As you relax yourself into this position, close your eyes. Allow your face, as well as your entire body, to be as relaxed and as at ease as possible. Breathe deeply and fully. If you would like to try it, this is a wonderful opportunity to practice the three-part yogic breathing presented in the "Pranayama" section of Chapter 16. Whether you practice this technique or not, allow your breathing to be full, deep, and rhythmic. Do not force the breath. Let your inhalation lead naturally to your exhalation, and back again to the following inhalation without pause. Abandon yourself. Surrender yourself into this position of total relaxation. Stay in this position as long as necessary.

Savasana is a wonderful pose to assume for a profoundly integrative, meditative, and restorative relaxation at the end of a yoga session. You will find instructions at the end of this Complete Yoga Session on how to perform *yoga nidra*, a deep yogic relaxation, while lying in savasana.

Complete Yoga Session: The Main Asanas

Once you've warmed up your body with the Sun Salutation and know how to rest if necessary during your session, you're ready to try the main poses of the Complete Yoga Session. The session continues with a sequence of standing postures, followed by an assortment of forward bends, backward bends, twisting poses, and inversions performed on the floor—all designed to give you a complete yoga workout for the entire body. Have fun as you continue your yoga session.

Trikonasana: Triangle Pose

Trikonasana, or "Triangle Pose," is a powerful asana that stretches and tones the entire body—arms, back, shoulders, groin area, and legs. It also stimulates the internal organs and

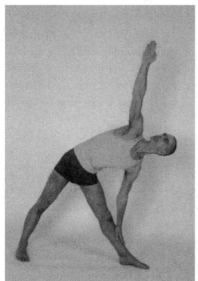

Fig. YPS.4a: Triangle Pose

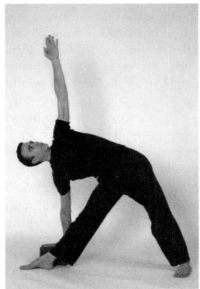

Fig. YPS.4b: Triangle Pose Supported With a Yoga Block

helps to promote proper body alignment, leading to increased grace and poise.

To prepare for Triangle Pose, stand in Mountain Pose. Mountain Pose is the opening position (page 114) for the Sun Salutation series: Your legs and feet are together, big toes touching and the rest of your toes spread out. With an exhalation, step or jump your feet about 3 to 4 feet apart as you raise your hands straight out to the sides at shoulder height, palms facing downward. Slide your left foot toward the left so that it is pointing directly in front of your left hip and forms a 90-degree angle to your body. Slide your right foot so that it is angled in toward your body at about a 30- to 45-degree angle. Your body is now facing toward the left and the heel of your right foot is directly in line with the center of your left foot. Inhale and shift your hips toward your left. As you exhale, shift your upper body toward the left. Lead with the fingers of the left hand as you pull yourself as far to the left as possible. Your arms are still parallel to the ground. When you've reached your maximum stretch to the left, lower your left hand to touch the left leg wherever it easily reaches—thigh, knee, shin, ankle, or foot. If you are extremely flexible, you may even be able touch the floor with your left fingertips or even the palm of your hand.

Keep both legs straight, knees gentle, but not bent. Rotate the right shoulder up toward the ceiling as you lift your right arm and hand straight up. Feel as though the movement is being initiated from the fingers of the raised right hand, as though they are being pulled toward the ceiling. Maintain as straight a position as possible—in the ideal posture, both your arms would form a single unbroken straight line perpendicular to the floor. Your torso would be perfectly parallel to both the floor and the wall in back or in front of you. This is the ideal. Accept where you and your body are today as you hold yourself in Triangle Pose for several breaths.

When you are ready to release from Triangle Pose, raise up your left arm on an exhalation while simultaneously lowering the right arm. Allow both arms to float down to your sides. Walk your feet back together again and rest for a few breaths in Mountain Pose. Take this time to breathe, relax, and center. Take stock of how you feel. Then prepare to perform Triangle Pose on the opposite side of your body.

If you have difficulty maintaining balance in the pose, try placing the palm of your hand on a support such as a wood or foam block. Fig. YPS.4b shows Triangle Pose toward the right side of the body with support from a yoga block.

Vrkasana: Tree Pose

Yoga helps to promote poise, grace, and balance. A group of postures known as balancing poses are especially helpful in achieving these goals. In addition to helping provide balance, these postures also help to promote concentration and clarity of thought because you must focus the mind with great awareness in order to balance the physical body.

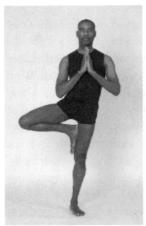

Fig. YPS.5a: Tree Pose With Hands at Center Breast

One of the best balancing postures is *vrkasana*, or "Tree Pose." In this posture, you balance yourself on one leg at a time while striving to achieve the rootedness and balance of a tree. This asana, in addition to promoting grace and balance, helps to stretch and tone the muscles of the legs and groin area. If you are new to Tree Pose or are still working to perfect this posture, you may want to position yourself next to a wall, chair, or table for added support as you try it.

To prepare for Tree Pose, stand erect in Mountain Pose. Slowly shift your body weight onto your left foot. Inhale as you raise your right leg and grasp your right foot with both hands. Flex your right leg so that your right knee points out to the right and your right inner thigh is facing directly forward in front of you. Place the sole of your right foot flat against your left inner thigh, knee, or ankle—as high up on your left leg as you comfortably can. The inside surface of your right thigh should be as parallel as possible to the wall in front of you. Press the little toe of the bent leg into the standing leg—this helps to release the hip of the bent leg and open the thigh even more. Both legs exert equal tension—the foot of the bent leg presses into the standing leg as the standing leg presses into the foot of the bent leg.

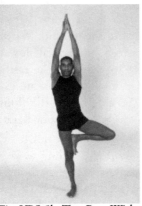

Fig. YPS.5b: Tree Pose With Arms Raised Overhead

Let your arms hang by your side for the time being. Take a few breaths as you steady yourself in Tree Pose. You will most likely find it easier to balance and maintain your placement in this posture if you fix your gaze steadily on one point located at or below eye level or on the floor in front of you.

If you find this posture challenging enough as you are now positioned, then simply hold this position for as long as you are able. If you feel stable in this position, then try raising your arms and hands into Prayer Position at the center of your chest (see Fig. YPS.5a). Hold and breathe several full breaths in this position. If you find this is challenging enough for you, then hold here for as long as you can. If you feel that you can go still further in Tree Pose, then slowly raise your arms up overhead. Check to make sure that your arms are straight and in line with your ears (see Fig. YPS.5b). If it is uncomfortable for you to bring your palms together—and for many men it is because of

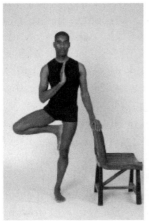

Fig. YPS.5c: Tree Pose With Chair Support

tightness in the shoulder area—then simply hold your arms pointing straight above your head toward the ceiling and parallel to one another. If you are accomplished in this posture, try closing your eyes.

When you are ready to release from Tree Pose, gently lower your arms to your sides as you release your bent leg to the floor. Breathe and relax. Take a moment to see how you feel, and then perform Tree Pose standing on the opposite leg.

If you find it difficult to maintain your balance in Tree Pose, try supporting yourself by placing your hands against a wall or on a table or chair. Fig. YPS.5c shows a modified version of Tree Pose with chair support. If necessary, lower the sole of the foot of the bent leg to the knee or ankle of the standing leg.

After you have performed Tree Pose on both sides of the body, take a moment to be aware of how you feel. Did you feel different from one side to the other as you performed Tree Pose?

Vrkasana can be a challenging posture. Work within your limits. Place the bent leg as far down on the standing leg as is necessary for you. Use a wall, chair, or other prop for support for as long as you need to. As you progress in your practice, Tree Pose should become easier for you. See if eventually you can execute Tree Pose with the eyes closed. As you gain greater dexterity and confidence in this pose, you may well find yourself gaining greater balance, poise, and clarity in many other areas of your life as well.

Paschimottanasana: Seated Forward Bend Pose

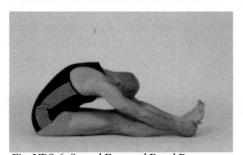

Fig. YPS.6: Seated Forward Bend Pose

Many men suffer from back pain—in particular, pain in the lower back. *Paschimottanasana*, commonly referred to as "Seated Forward Bend Pose," is one of the best asanas that you can perform to help relieve back pain, especially lower back pain. Back pain is often caused by tight hamstring muscles, an important muscle group that runs along the entire length of the backs of the thighs. For many men, the hamstrings are among the tightest (that is, most contracted) muscles in the body. Seated Forward Bend Pose helps to relax and stretch the muscles all along the entire length of the spine and the backs of the legs. When properly performed, it is an excellent pose for sciatica. In addition, it helps to stimulate the organs in the abdominal cavity, thus promoting digestion and elimination.

Come to a seated position on the floor with your legs straight out in front of you, parallel to one another. Sit on your buttocks with your upper body in a 90-degree angle to the floor. If this position is uncomfortable for you, place a blanket or folded towel under your sit-bones. Make sure that your buttocks are securely resting on the floor or the padded support you've selected. Use your hands to grasp the flesh of your buttocks to pull the fleshy tissue away from your sit-bones. Feel that your sit-bones are resting firmly on the floor. To increase your preparedness for the posture, press the palms of your hands directly on the floor outside of your buttocks as you lift your back and head up into a straight vertical position.

As you inhale, lift your arms overhead, parallel to one another and in line with your ears. As you exhale, slowly hinge forward from the groin. Do your best not to round or arch your back, and don't try to touch your feet or legs yet. Maintain your stretch in this position for several breaths. Deepen the stretch by folding from the hip joints. Feel as though your groin area and the creases between the pelvis and your hips form a hinge and your torso is folding forward from this hinge. Keep your back as straight as possible as you fold and reach forward. Feel as though someone is pulling on your fingertips, lengthening your entire back.

On an exhalation, allow your body to fold completely forward. Use your hands to grasp your heels, toes, balls of your feet, arches of the feet, ankles, shins, or even just your knees or thighs—wherever you are able to reach most comfortably. Maintain this full stretch for several complete deep breaths. With each inhalation, feel yourself lengthening forward. With each exhalation, feel your torso coming even closer to your legs. Be kind and understanding to yourself. Accept your body wherever it may be in terms of flexibility and stretching capacity. With practice, your stretch should deepen even further. With each breath, feel life and energy circulating into your back, legs, and throughout your entire body. If you feel any areas of particular tension or holding, allow your breath to travel there. To help support you in this pose, you might try wrapping a belt, strap, or towel around your feet and holding the strap or whatever support you've chosen with both your hands to stretch forward more comfortably.

Paschimottanasana is often referred to as a pose of surrender. Allow yourself to surrender and release. Let go. Let go of any holding you may have—especially in your lower back. In Asian thought, the back is associated with the West, which represents our past. Paschimottanasana literally means "Intense Stretch of the West." Often, in the tension we carry in our backs we are carrying a lifetime of physical and psychological traumas. Let go of whatever you are holding onto. Abandon yourself into the pose.

To come out of Seated Forward Bend Pose, raise your upper body up away from your thighs as you straighten your arms and raise them overhead. Come back to sit securely on your sit-bones as you release your arms down alongside your body.

Close your eyes and take a few moments to feel the effects that Seated Forward Bend Pose has had on you—body, mind, and spirit.

Janu Sirsasana: Head-to-Knee Pose

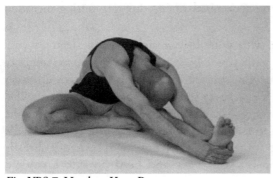

Fig. YPS.7: Head-to-Knee Pose

The next asana, *janu sirsasana*, or "Head-to-Knee Pose," also helps to stretch out the spine and the backs of the legs while giving an added stretch to the groin and hip area. It can be helpful to practice janu sirsasana once the body has been warmed and stretched by Seated Forward Bend Pose.

Remain in a seated position on the floor with your legs extended out in front of you, as you did above in preparation for Seated

Forward Bend Pose. Bend your right leg and place the heel of your right foot as close to the genital area as you can. The sole of your right foot rests against your left inner thigh, or however high you are able to place it against your left leg. Your right knee is as close to the ground as possible. Your right lower leg forms a right angle to your left leg. If your right knee does not touch the floor, you can support it by placing a pillow, folded towel, or blanket under it.

Place your hands on your left thigh and use your hands to help rotate your torso around to your left so that the midline of your torso is placed as directly above the midline of the left thigh as possible. The foot of your left leg is flexed and the midline of your left thigh is facing directly toward the ceiling.

On an inhalation, raise your arms up over your head. Your inner arms are parallel to your head and in line with the ears. On an exhalation, fold forward from the hips as you position your upper body directly over the midline of your left thigh. Try to position your torso parallel over your thigh. With your hands, grasp the heel, sole, toes, or ball of your left foot, or your left ankle, shin, knee, or thigh—wherever you are able to reach comfortably. (See Fig. YPS.7.) Try not to round your torso forward. Rather, fold from the hip creases and let your back remain as straight and extended as possible. To help support you in this pose, you may want to try wrapping a belt, strap, or towel around your left foot and hold it with both hands.

Hold this position for several breaths. Feel the entire back of your spine lengthening and your right hip area opening. To increase the stretch in your right hip, you might experiment with pressing down on your right thigh with your right hand. Apply gentle, but firm, pressure above the knee. Avoid pressing directly on the knee itself. Do not add this refinement if you have any knee or hip concerns, or if the variation is uncomfortable in any way. Feel your entire hip and groin area opening, releasing, and widening as you hold this position.

When you are ready to come out of the position, inhale as you raise your torso up from your thigh, initiating your movements with the head and upper chest. Allow your arms and hands to come gently back to your sides. Release your right leg, extending it forward in front of you. Wiggle it from side to side and allow it to come back in line with your straight, extended left leg.

Repeat Head-to-Knee Pose on the opposite side of your body.

Bhujangasana: Cobra Pose

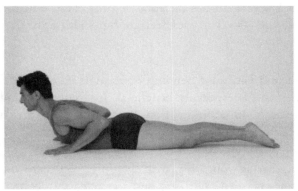

Fig. YPS.8: Cobra Pose

Bhujangasana, or "Cobra Pose," introduces the first of two backward bending yoga postures. Many men today tend to have hunched shoulders that round forward. Sitting for long hours at desks, in front of computers, or at the steering wheel of a car; working hard at the gym to develop strong pectoral, or chest, muscles; genetic predisposition; and the effect of aging on the musculoskeletal system are all factors that contribute to creating and aggravating this situation. Backward bending exercises are an ideal way to strengthen the muscles of the back in order to compensate for the weakness that often exists in the back and shoulder areas.

Yoga aims systematically to balance all the muscles in the body. Hence, postures that stretch and tone one group of muscles are generally followed by postures that stretch and tone the muscles that are opposite in action. The backward bending exercises that follow are the perfect counterpostures to the forward bending postures you've just performed. As always, listen to your body. If you feel that this or any of the following backward bending exercises are causing you discomfort, skip them, and rest in Child's or Corpse Pose.

Cobra Pose is especially good for strengthening the muscles of the upper back and opening the shoulders. Lie down flat on your belly on a mat or on a comfortable padded surface. Your legs and feet should be close together and in contact with the floor. Your toes are pointed and the tops of your feet are in contact with the ground. Place your hands, palms flat on the ground, underneath each of your respective shoulders. The arms should be bent with the elbows close to the sides of your body and the upper arms parallel to the floor. Your chin should be flat on the ground.

With an inhalation, slowly begin to inch your chin forward and up. Direct the forward upward movement from the sternum, chest, and heart center so that the head and neck stay in alignment with the rest of the spine. Gently continue to lift your neck, upper back, middle back, and lower back forward and up as each vertebra of your spine draws upward. Keep your hands on the floor. Use the strength of your back, especially your upper back, to propel your torso upward. Do not push on your hands to do the work, use them only to stabilize yourself in the posture. If you can, arch your neck and look up and backward. Go only so far as you are able. Feel as though you are a cobra, rising slowly, vertebra by vertebra as you strengthen the muscles of your entire back. Feel this movement extending all the way to your tailbone. Hold this position several breaths or longer if it is comfortable. When you are ready to release, gently return to the beginning position, chin on the floor, with a slow exhalation.

Repeat Cobra Pose up to three times if you are just beginning your yoga program. With continued practice, you can try increasing the length of time that you hold each repetition of the posture, as well as the number of repetitions that you can do.

If you find that performing Cobra Pose is too challenging for you, try modifying the pose. Experiment with placing your hands several inches in front of your chest. You can also try spreading your legs wider behind you—so that your feet are hip-width apart.

Dhanurasana: Bow Pose

Dhanurasana, or "Bow Pose," is a second backward bending exercise. It is one of the most frequently performed yoga exercises and is especially beneficial. It strengthens and invigorates both the legs and the entire back. In addition, Bow Pose helps bring a rich supply of blood to the abdominal area, resulting in a healing and restorative effect on all the internal organs, and, in particular, the digestive organs.

To prepare for Bow Pose, remain lying flat on your belly, with the tip of your nose and your chin resting on the floor. Your toes are pointed. Your legs and feet remain in contact with the ground, but you can now spread them apart so that your feet are about hip-width distance apart. Bend your legs so that your lower legs form a 90-degree angle to the ground. Reach back with your hands and securely grasp the shin of each leg with the corresponding hand. If it is too challenging to hold on to the shins, then try holding on to the ankles. Using your hands, press each foot as close to the outer hip (the outside of the buttocks) as possible. Hold.

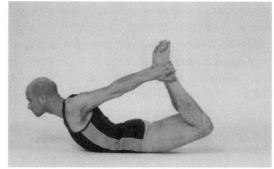

Fig. YPS.9: Bow Pose

With an inhalation, gently begin to draw your quadriceps off the ground. Lift your thighs as high off the floor as possible. Slowly begin to lift the chest forward and up off the floor as your torso arches backward. The thighs lift, the knees lift, and the heels lift from the buttocks. Press the shins away from the head to open the shoulders and back. Be careful not to strain your neck by arching it too far back. Feel your belly fully positioned on the floor. You are becoming a bow. Feel the rich supply of blood that is rushing to your abdominal area as you practice Bow Pose.

Hold Bow Pose for as long as is comfortable for you. When you are ready to release your body from the posture, exhale and slowly release your upper body, arms, and legs to the floor. Let your legs and feet float back to the floor and turn your head to one side. Rest and relax for several breaths. When you are ready, repeat Bow Pose one or two times more.

You may find Bow Pose challenging. If you are a beginner, it may help for you to spread your knees wide apart. As you progress in the pose, try bringing your legs closer together until your knees eventually touch.

Ardha Matsyendrasana: Seated Spinal Twist

You have done a very powerful yoga practice. Congratulate yourself on your progress through this yoga session. Breathe, relax, and center yourself for the practice yet to follow.

You have performed an impressive warm-up and overall conditioning round of exercises in the Sun Salutation series. You have helped increase flexibility to your spine while strengthening your back and bathing your spinal column and nerves in oxygen-rich blood with standing and balancing poses and forward and backward bends.

You are now ready to perform a powerful twisting posture. Twisting movements help bring greater mobility to the sides of the body. Backward and forward bending postures help develop strength and flexibility in extending and flexing the spine up and down. Spinal twisting postures help to increase the ability to rotate the torso laterally, helping to strengthen the muscles on the sides of the spine and the

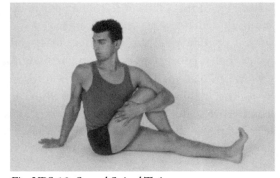

Fig. YPS.10: Seated Spinal Twist

rest of the torso. In addition, when we perform twisting movements, we "squeeze" our internal organs, massaging them from the inside out. This helps to stimulate all of our internal organs, assisting to cleanse them of toxins that may have built up and promoting optimum functioning of such important organs as the liver, kidneys, lungs, and spleen—not to mention our organs of digestion and elimination. So, have fun as you twist and turn your way to better health the yoga way.

Ardha matsyendrasana literally means "Half Lord of the Fishes Pose," and is often referred to simply as "Seated Spinal Twist." This pose is a comfortable way to provide a complete and potent twist to the entire body. To prepare for this twist, assume a comfortable seated position on your mat or on a padded surface. Hold your torso, neck, and head erect, with your legs straight out in front of you and touching. Your arms are straight out at your sides, palms pressing down into the floor at the sides of the hips to help you achieve as erect a posture as possible. Leaving the left leg stretched out straight in front of you, bend the right leg at the knee and place the sole of the right foot firmly on the ground outside the left knee. Your right knee is flexed and your right leg forms an inverted V shape relative to the floor. If you are a beginner, hug your right leg around the area of the knee with your left arm (see Fig. YPS.10). If this position is easy for you, or if you are more advanced in your yoga practice, try moving your left arm and hand so that your left upper arm is on the outside of your right thigh. Grasp the shin, calf, or knee—whichever you are able to—with your left hand. Check the alignment of your spine, and if necessary, adjust your placement so that your torso, neck, and head remain as straight and erect as possible. As you inhale, take your right arm and place the palm or fingertips of your right hand on the floor behind you as you twist gently, but firmly, to your right. Try to place your right arm and hand in line with the spine. Keep your head erect and turn your neck to look as far behind you to the right as you comfortably can. Breathe fully and deeply in complete respirations. With each inhalation, lift your spine higher; with each exhalation, twist a little further to the right.

Continue to breathe fully and deeply as you maintain your body in this powerful spinal twist. To help you achieve the maximum twist, try adjusting your position by rotating your right shoulder to twist it back and around even a little more toward the right. Press into your right hand to help stabilize you. Feel the twist originating all the way down from the base of the spine and the lower abdomen. The lower vertebrae of the spine have less flexibility in rotating to the side than they do in bending forward and back; take advantage of this position to rotate your lower torso as far to the side as possible. Allow your stomach and the other internal organs in the solar plexus to twist even further to the right as you provide a deep, compressing massage to your internal organs: They are quite literally your vital organs, responsible for maintaining your health and vitality.

When you are ready to release from this twist, exhale and gently release your body back to center. Allow yourself to rotate your torso past center and a little to your left as a countertwist, and then come back to center. Release your right leg back to the floor. Take a few moments to breathe, center, and relax. Then repeat the asana on the other side of your body by executing a spinal twist to your left.

When you have performed Seated Spinal Twist on both sides of the body, lower your back, neck, and head to the floor. If you feel a need to rest, stretch your legs out in front of you and assume Corpse Pose. Take time to breathe, center, and relax.

Setu Bandha Sarvangasana: Bridge Pose

Setu bandha sarvangasana, or "Bridge Pose," is a particularly enjoyable and relaxing backward bending exercise. It gives a good stretch to the chest, neck, and spine, and helps to open the pelvis, groin, and hip area. It brings a fresh supply of richly oxygenated blood to the legs and lungs, rejuvenating tired legs and helping to relieve chest problems such as congestion and breathing disorders.

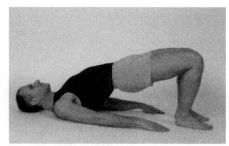

Fig. YPS.11: Bridge Pose

To prepare for Bridge Pose, lie flat on your back with your arms alongside your body a few inches away from each side of the torso, palms facing down. Bend your legs and bring the heels of your feet as close to the buttocks as possible, your feet parallel to one another or slightly pigeon-toed (the toes of the feet pointing slightly inward).

As you exhale, press your feet and arms into the ground as you lift the pelvis off the floor. Lift the buttocks as you peel them off the floor. Open the front hip creases. Gradually lift your back off the floor as you lift your buttocks higher. Unstack your vertebrae from the floor—one by one—beginning with those at the base of the spine and progressing up to the very top of the shoulders. As your upper back lifts off the floor, try to press your shoulders closer to the ground by sliding your hands under your back. If this pose is easy and comfortable for you so far, try going deeper in the pose by grasping your palms together under your back on the floor and interlacing your fingers. Rock your upper back gently from side to side to allow you to press your shoulder blades closer together. If this refinement is too challenging for you, then let your arms rest firmly on the floor in front of you, as illustrated in Fig. YPS.11.

Hold Bridge Pose for several breaths. Feel an entire wave of relaxation spreading down your back as it widens and opens—all the way from the top of the shoulders to the base of the spine. When you are ready to release your body from Bridge Pose, exhale and gently release your spine and buttocks to the floor, beginning at the shoulders and moving down to the middle back, the lower back, and finally the buttocks. Repeat Bridge Pose one or two more times. When you have finished with Bridge Pose, unbend your knees and straighten your legs as you allow them to return back down to the floor, spread out about hip-width apart. Roll your legs from side to side. Rest and relax. Take a moment to register how you feel after having completed Bridge Pose.

Take a moment to remind yourself of what a good job you are doing. You are helping your back to remain healthy and stress-free with this basic yet complete series of yoga postures.

Sarvangasana: Shoulderstand

Sarvangasana, popularly known as "Shoulderstand," is an inverted pose. Inverted postures (also referred to as inversions) are those in which the head is placed in a position

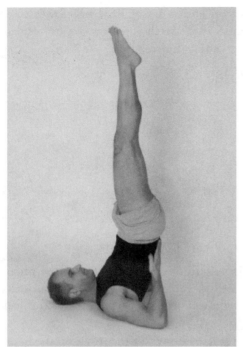

Fig. YPS.12: Shoulderstand

below the heart. Inversions are particularly powerful ways to counterbalance the effect of gravity on the body. When the head is placed below the heart, the brain receives an extremely rich supply of blood. At the same time, the internal organs are allowed some measure of release from their usual positions as they are suspended in a reverse direction. This helps to provide them with both added stimulation and rest.

In sarvangasana, you lie on the floor on your back and raise your legs in a vertical line up above you in a Shoulderstand position. *Sarvangasana* literally means "Whole Body Pose," and, indeed, it engages and benefits the whole body. This asana is referred to as the "queen of yoga postures" because of its many excellent benefits. It helps to improve circulation, calm the nervous system, and aid all the internal organs. It is said to have a very beneficial effect on the functioning of the thyroid gland, which is an essential organ in regulating many of the body's functions.

To prepare for Shoulderstand, lie flat on your back on your mat or on a comfortable padded surface. Your arms are stretched out along the sides of the body, palms facing down and fingers touching the floor.

As you inhale, bend your legs and slowly lift them off the ground. Allow your knees to come above your forehead. Slowly raise your legs up above you. If you need to assist your legs with helping hands, do so. Your torso and legs should form a vertical line to the floor. Your feet are neither pointed nor flexed, but neutral. To maintain your thighs and lower legs in a straight, neutral position, you can point your toes inward a bit—pigeon-toed—so that your big toes are touching. Bend your arms, with your upper arms and elbows resting on the floor as close to the body as possible. Place the palms of your two hands on your back, alongside and parallel to the spine and as close to the shoulder blades as possible. This will give you support in Shoulderstand. The closer your shoulders are to the ground, the better. To achieve a better position, draw the tops of your shoulders underneath you. Press your chest to your chin. Your weight should be resting on your elbows and shoulders. Lift the back of your body so that the back, buttocks, legs, and heels are lifting as vertically as possible.

Continue to breathe normally as you maintain Shoulderstand. When you are ready to release from Shoulderstand, you can come out of the pose in either of two ways. If you'd like to release completely from Shoulderstand, then simply roll out of the pose: Return your arms alongside your body, palms facing down. Using your arms and hands for support, gently unroll your back and spine, vertebra by vertebra. If necessary, bend your knees as you do so in order to relieve any strain on your back. Return your legs to the floor, spread roughly hip-width apart, arms slightly out to the sides, and relax for a few breaths.

If you would like to continue to flow into the next posture, *halasana*, or "Plow Pose," then do so by following the next set of directions.

When first beginning to do Shoulderstand, try holding the posture for as long as is comfortable, even if it is only for a few seconds. With practice, you will gain confidence and mastery. Eventually, see if you can hold this position for several minutes.

If you find that doing Shoulderstand is a strain, you can try practicing an alternate inversion, "Legs-up-the-Wall Pose," where the legs rest against the wall for support. (See Fig. 13.3 on page 164.)

Once you've practiced Shoulderstand, take the opportunity to see how you feel, both during your practice and in the time that follows your practice. Shoulderstand is an inverted posture, and your body is quite literally "upside-down," with your head on the ground and your feet pointing upward in the air. This pose just might make you see your world—in ever so subtle a way—just a little bit differently.

Please note: The Shoulderstand is one of the most highly touted postures in yoga practice. It can benefit nearly everyone. Because of the inverted position, however, it can increase the flow of blood, especially to the head. For this reason, it is not recommended for people with heart problems (especially high blood pressure), glaucoma or other eye disorders, and anyone with neck injuries or problems. For any female readers, it is also contraindicated for menstruating or pregnant women. As with any yoga posture, please check with your doctor before practicing if you have any particular health concern.

Halasana: Plow Pose

Halasana, or "Plow Pose," is frequently practiced in a seamless flow following the Shoulderstand. It helps to further open the shoulders and spine, promotes the proper functioning of the thyroid gland, and can help to improve overall circulation.

It's easy to flow into Plow Pose directly from Shoulderstand. When you're ready to release from Shoulderstand, slowly lower your legs and feet beyond your head as far back as you can reach and as close to the ground as possible. Try to keep your legs straight. If your feet don't touch the ground, that's alright. If possible, keep your arms in their original position, pointing forward in front of the body, palms pressing into the ground (see Fig. YPS.13a). Feel the nice stretch that you're giving to the entire back. If you can, touch the floor above your head with the balls of your toes. Flex your feet so that the toes are curled under and pointing as directly toward the head as possible

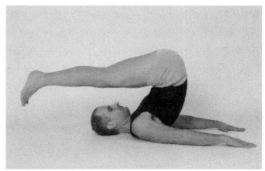

Fig. YPS.13a: Plow Pose With Legs Parallel to the Floor

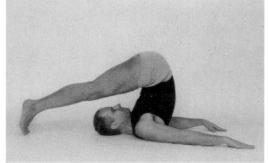

Fig. YPS.13b: Plow Pose With Toes Touching the Floor

(see Fig. YPS.13b). If it's easy for you to touch the ground with your feet, try spreading your legs out to the side in a straddle, still keeping them straight. Bring your legs and feet back together again. Bend your legs and see if you can rest your knees on or slightly above your ears. If you're extremely flexible in this position, try wrapping your arms around the backs of the thighs. For an easier variation of Plow Pose, gently rest your knees on your forehead without trying to straighten them out beyond your head.

When you are ready to release from Plow Pose, press down on your arms and hands, slowly raise your feet overhead, and then allow your torso to roll back down to the floor vertebra by vertebra, bending your knees if necessary to protect your back. Rest and relax for a few breaths if you feel the need.

As an additional variation of Shoulderstand, you can also assume Plow Pose as a preparatory step before rising to full Shoulderstand. From the starting position for Shoulderstand, lying flat on your back on the floor, gently raise your legs overhead and beyond your head. See if you can touch the floor beyond your head with the balls of your feet. Then slowly raise your legs up to a 90-degree angle to the floor, tips of the toes in line with your forehead, for Shoulderstand.

If you would like to practice Plow Pose as a posture independent of the Shoulderstand, it's easy to do that, too. Just assume the base position for preparing for the Shoulderstand: lie flat on your back, arms out to the sides, palms facing down. Slowly bend your legs and lift your legs overhead, pressing down on your hands and arms for support. Lift your legs up and over your head so that they are pointing beyond and away from the head. Keep your legs as straight as possible and reach as far back behind you as you can with your feet as close to the ground as possible. Experiment with any of the variations you wish while in Plow Pose.

When you are ready to release from Plow Pose, press down on your arms and hands, slowly raise your feet and legs overhead, and roll your upper body down vertebra by vertebra, bending your knees if necessary to protect your back. As a counterpose to Shoulderstand and Plow Pose, come immediately into Fish Pose to ease any tightness in the back.

Matsyasana: Fish Pose

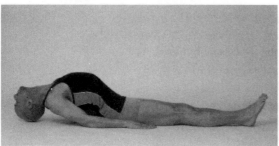

Fig. YPS.14: Fish Pose

Matsyasana, or "Fish Pose," is nearly always recommended as a counterposture to Shoulderstand. A typical sequencing in a basic yoga session includes Bridge Pose followed by Shoulderstand, which flows into Plow Pose, and is followed by Fish Pose. Fish Pose provides a strong stretch to the chest area, allowing it to expand and fill with oxygen in a way virtually unparalleled by any other exercise, yogic or otherwise.

To prepare for Fish Pose, bring your legs and feet together while lying on your back. Place your arms close alongside your body, palms facing down just outside of your hips. Gently bending your upper arms and pressing onto your elbows, exhale and lift between the shoulder blades as your chest forms an upward arch. Let the top of your head rest on the floor. Take several deep breaths in this position. Feel your lungs and rib cage expand as you experience the rich benefits of Fish Pose. Allow the weight of your upper body to be supported primarily by your elbows and only secondarily by your head. When you're ready to release from Fish Pose, exhale as you gently lower your back onto the floor.

If you are just beginning to practice Fish Pose, try holding the asana for several breaths. With practice, see if you can hold the position for several minutes. You may find it more comfortable to place a folded towel or pillow under your head as your perform this asana.

Oxygen is the fuel that the body uses to accomplish virtually all of its activities. By performing Fish Pose, you are filling up your lungs with an extraordinarily rich supply of oxygen. After you've practiced this pose, take a few moments to see how you feel. Do you feel like a fish floating on your back in water? Are you more invigorated? Energized? As your day progresses, see if you notice any difference in your energy levels and breathing patterns.

Yoga Nidra: Deep Relaxation

Many yoga classes conclude with what is known as *yoga nidra*, which literally means "yoga sleep." Yoga nidra is more commonly known as "Deep Relaxation," or when performed at the end of a yoga session, "Final Relaxation." This deeply calming experience can help you to integrate the benefits achieved during your yoga session, as well as let go of any areas where you may still be holding tension—whether that tension be physical, mental, emotional, or even spiritual. Nearly every yoga class concludes with a period of deep relaxation. Many yoga teachers believe that this is the most important part of a yoga practice. It provides the opportunity not only to integrate the benefits of your yoga session, but also to tune in to yourself—a priceless benefit for the typical man suffering from the pressures of time constraints and societal demands.

There are many powerful ways of preparing for Deep Relaxation. The relaxation exercise that follows was inspired by my recollection of one very deep and restorative yoga session I enjoyed with a teacher at the Sivananda Yoga Vedanta Center in New York City. Try concluding your yoga practice session with this progressive relaxation exercise. I suggest that you read through the following instructions in their entirety before you try the relaxation so that you'll have an understanding of the overall procedure. You may find it helpful to have someone read you the instructions as you follow along and relax. Another helpful way to use this relaxation exercise is for you to make a tape recording of the instructions as you read them through slowly, then play back the tape as you follow the instructions for the relaxation.

While Deep Relaxation is frequently performed at the end of a yoga session, you can perform yoga nidra any time you are in need of relaxation, independent of practicing other yoga poses. Assuming yoga nidra when you come home from work can be deeply restorative.

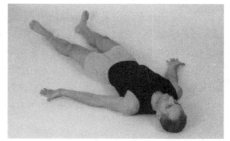

Final Relaxation Exercise

Lie down on the floor, preferably on a carpet or other padded surface, with your back resting on the

Fig. YPS.15: Final Relaxation

floor in Corpse Pose. The backs of the legs should be resting firmly on the floor, your two legs spread slightly apart—hip-width or perhaps a little wider. The backs of your arms should be resting securely on the ground, with your arms spread slightly apart from your body, your palms facing up.

You are now ready to do a nice, long relaxation. This relaxation will allow you to integrate all the benefits of the yoga session that you have just been doing, as well as to release any toxins and tension from your body. First, you'll begin with a physical relaxation, followed by a mental relaxation, for a complete relaxation of body, mind, and soul.

Extend your right leg out in front of you. Pick it up off the ground. Squeeze it tightly. Now release it.

Extend your left leg out in front of you. Pick it up off the ground. Squeeze it tightly. Now release it.

Gently roll your legs from side to side and let them slowly come to a comfortable position as they spread out slightly away from the midline of the body.

Now pick your buttocks up off the ground. Squeeze them. Release them.

Lift your shoulders up high toward your head. Now lower them down completely toward your feet. Now relax your shoulders.

Extend your right arm long alongside your body. Pick it up off the floor. Squeeze it tightly. Make a fist out of your right hand. Hold—tighter, tighter, tighter. Now let go of your arm. Release it to the floor and allow it to relax.

Extend your left arm long alongside your body. Pick it up off the floor. Squeeze it tightly. Make a fist out of your left hand. Hold—tighter, tighter, tighter. Now let go of your arm. Release it to the floor and allow it to relax.

Gently roll your arms from side to side and let them slowly come to a comfortable position as they spread out slightly away from the midline of the body. Let your fingers be open and relaxed.

Squeeze your face. Make it into a prune. Stick out your tongue. Crinkle your nose up into a tight ball. Now release your entire face and relax it.

Take some time now to travel back up through your body from the toes of your feet to the top of your head as you release any residual tension that you may still be harboring.

Bring your awareness to your feet. Say to yourself, "My feet, ankles, and heels feel warm and heavy and are relaxing. My feet, ankles, and heels are completely relaxed. My calves, knees, and thighs feel warm and heavy and are relaxing. My calves, knees, and thighs are completely relaxed."

Now bring your consciousness to the hips, the buttocks, the pelvis, and the organs of the pelvis. Say, "My hips, buttocks, and pelvis feel warm and heavy and are relaxing. My hips, buttocks, and pelvis are completely relaxed."

Bring your awareness to your back, spine, and torso. Say, "My spine and back feel heavy and warm and are relaxing. My spine and back are completely relaxed. My abdomen, torso, and chest feel heavy and warm and are relaxing. My abdomen, torso, and chest are completely relaxed."

Bring your awareness to your shoulders, arms, hands, and fingers. Say, "My shoulders, arms, hands, and fingers feel heavy and warm and are relaxing. My shoulders, arms, hands, and fingers are completely relaxed."

Now bring your awareness to your neck and head. Say, "My neck, jaw, chin, mouth, cheeks, eyes, forehead, back of my head, and scalp feel warm and heavy. My neck, jaw, chin, mouth, cheeks, eyes, forehead, back of my head, and scalp are completely relaxed."

Now bring your awareness to the internal organs of the body. Say, "My intestines, stomach, pancreas, liver, lungs, kidneys, and even my brain feel warm and heavy and are relaxing. My intestines, stomach, pancreas, liver, lungs, kidneys, and even my brain are completely relaxed. My entire being—body, mind, and soul—is completely relaxed."

Yoga nidra is a time for deep surrender. Allow yourself to surrender completely as you absorb and integrate all the benefits of the postures you have been performing.

Allow your breathing to be full, deep, and relaxed. Enjoy the blissful sensation of peace and calm as you allow yourself to surrender your body, mind, and soul. You have nothing to do—only to be. Just be, in this present moment. Be receptive to the healing power of the life force that is flowing through you with each breath that you take. Be grateful for the restorative and energizing power of this relaxation exercise and of all of your yoga practice.

Yoga nidra affords us the opportunity to be not only physically relaxed, but also more mentally aware. Take a moment to register your awareness of how you feel. Do you feel differently now than when you first lay down to begin the relaxation exercise? If you have just finished practicing the yoga postures, do you feel differently than you did before you began your yoga today? Does your body feel lighter? Heavier? Denser? Are you aware of any areas of opening? Or any areas where you might still be holding? How does your breath feel to you? Is it deep, calm, and relaxed? Or short and irregular? Do any visual images or auditory or tactile impressions arise? Are you falling asleep? Register your awareness of any sensations that you may be experiencing. Note them, and let them go.

Allow yourself to remain in this restorative and meditative final relaxation posture for as long as you wish.

When you are ready to return to the here and now, do so slowly and mindfully. Begin to bring your awareness back to your breathing. Take a deep, full inhalation and a deep exhalation. Wiggle your fingers and toes gently. Stretch your arms up over your head and out on the floor above your head. Stretch out your legs and arms, giving you a nice stretch from head to toe. Gently open your eyes. Feel as though you are waking up and stretching as you would in the morning after a good night's rest. Imagine what an infant feels like as it stretches out after a peaceful nap. Hug your knees up to your chest. Roll your knees from side to side. Then gently roll over onto one side in a fetal position. Supporting yourself with your hand and arm, slowly come back up to a sitting position.

Take the time to thank yourself for allowing yourself to do this stress-reducing and energizing yoga practice today. Thank yourself for giving yourself the gift of this relaxation. You're on the road to yoga health and well-being. Keep up your journey!

Creating Your Personal Yoga Practice Session

If you are just beginning to practice yoga, try performing the Complete Yoga Session presented here a number of times so that you become familiar with and feel easy in each pose. Once you've practiced for a period of time, you can try adapting the session to meet your own personal needs.

Yoga poses are commonly categorized into several key groups depending upon the major movement that is generated by the posture—thus, most yoga asanas are classified as backward bends, forward bends, balancing poses, inversions, or twists. If your goal is to get a complete body workout, try incorporating at least one posture from each group of exercises. You could adapt the Complete Yoga Session to a shorter practice time by performing one complete round of Sun Salutation, one forward bend (Head-to-Knee Posture), one backward bend (Cobra, Bow, or Bridge Pose), a balancing pose (Tree Pose), an inversion (Shoulderstand or Plow Pose), and a twist (Seated Spinal Twist). If you decide to practice an abbreviated program on a more regular basis, see if you can vary the pose you choose from each group in each session or each week (for instance, alternating Cobra with Bow Pose as your backward bending exercise).

If your time is really limited, you may want to do several rounds of the Sun Salutation—this powerful series of movements was designed to stretch and strengthen the entire body. If you are concerned about one particular area—for example, opening up the chest—you might want to focus on doing backward bending exercises. If you have tight hamstring and lower back muscles, you may want to focus on forward bending exercises. Remember, though, that it is always best to balance one type of posture by its opposite—for instance, a forward bend by a backward bend.

In addition to the asanas provided in "A Complete Yoga Practice Session for Men," you'll find various additional postures presented in the chapters in this book that are devoted to a man's specific needs. Try incorporating some of these poses into your yoga routine as you gain more experience and confidence with yoga.

This Complete Yoga Session is intended for fit men in good physical condition. The particular manner in which you pursue your yoga practice will depend upon your age and physical condition. If you are young and energetic, you may want to practice all the poses regularly and with a number of repetitions of each pose. If you're older or not so physically fit, you may want to start off gently, with only some of the poses and modifying them to your abilities, with fewer repetitions. With time and disciplined practice, though, you should be able to increase your stamina in your yoga practice, whatever your starting point.

When developing your yoga practice, regular practice is invaluable. If possible, see if you can incorporate a one-hour yoga practice session two to three times a week into your routine. If that proves too much, see if you can practice yoga for one hour once a week, or three times a week for a 20-minute session each time. It is better to choose fewer postures and perform them with awareness than to try to cram a lot of postures into a short time period. The benefits of yoga come with time—so if you're just beginning your yoga practice, try to commit yourself to a regular practice. Even if you may not feel the benefits after the first or second session, make a contract with yourself to continue for a stated period of time—at least four to six weeks—to give yoga the opportunity to have its effect on you. Chances are you'll be glad you did.

As you progress in your yoga practice, remember that yoga is more than just about physical exercise. It can also help promote the health and vitality of the mind, emotions, and spirit. Consider incorporating meditation and breathing practices into your yoga program for a complete yoga workout. You'll find more information on these practices in Chapter 16.

PART IV

YOGA FOR A MAN'S SPECIAL NEEDS

While yoga can help everyone—both men and women—there are special, important ways in which it can help today's man. The following chapters show you how yoga can be a vital part of your own health and wellness program, no matter how old (or young!) you are. You'll learn how yoga can meet the special needs of your stage in life, how it can enhance your athletic and fitness activities, address common health concerns specific to men, enhance your sex life, and even be practiced in pairs or groups.

Chapter 11

YOGA FOR THE PHASES
OF A MAN'S LIFE

Everyone can begin (yoga), and the point at which we start is very personal, and individual depending on where we are at the time.[1]

—T.K.V. Desikachar

Yoga is for every man. It is not only for men with perfect bodies in perfect shape. It is for young men, old men, in-shape men, and out-of-shape men. Indeed, yoga recognizes that there is no perfect body and no perfect shape—we are all, each and every one of us, perfect as we are, and realizing our perfection in different ways at different phases of our lives. The practice of yoga is a process of growth and development that can help take you from where you are now to the next stage of your journey—with grace, strength, confidence, and inner joy.

Yoga has developed ways of working with men of all ages and physical backgrounds and needs. No matter what your age or physical state may be at the moment, there is a style of yoga to suit you. The following are just some of the ways in which yoga can be helpful to you—wherever you are in your life journey.

Yoga and a Man's Life Passages

Men have different needs—physically, emotionally, mentally, and spiritually—at different phases in their lives. Many books have been written on the various stages and passages in a man's life by such well-known authors as Gail Sheehey (*Understanding Men's Passages*) and James Wilder (*Life Passages for Men*). The yoga tradition also recognizes that

143

men have different needs at different periods in their lives, and has developed ways of helping men make the most of each phase of life, while preparing them to make the transition to the next step in their journey.

One of the most influential of all yoga teachers was the South Indian yoga master teacher, Krishnamacharya (1888–1989). It is thanks to his search early in the 20th century to find the authentic sources of hatha yoga that most yoga practitioners today owe their practice. In search for authentic hatha yoga training, he traveled to the sacred caves of Nepal to study with one of the few remaining hatha yoga adepts at the sacred temple of Sringeri Math. The tradition that formed the basis for his approach to yoga is traced back to the revered sage Nathamuni (circa 800 C.E.), and through him, to the earliest recorded authority on yoga, Patanjali (circa 200 to 500 C.E.).

Krishnamacharya is responsible for expanding these sacred, traditional practices beyond their limited exercise by a few priestly (male only at the time) initiates and making them available to laypeople—men and women alike. He directly taught these practices to many of the most influential and well-known teachers of yoga in India—teachers who eventually developed their own schools of yoga and exported hatha yoga practices to the United States. Notable among these teachers are B.K.S. Iyengar, perhaps the most well-known teacher of yoga in the West (see Chapter 4); Pattabhi Jois (see Chapter 6); as well as his own son, T.K.V. Desikachar, who has trained many influential yoga practitioners and teachers. Another great teacher of yoga whose work has been widely disseminated in the West, Swami Sivananda (see Chapter 5), also traces his lineage to the same sacred temple of Sringeri Math.[2] The yoga tradition from which these practices that form the substratum of most yoga that is practiced in the United States today acknowledged from the very beginning that yoga should be adapted to suit the needs of the individual who was practicing it. And that meant different emphases for people of different ages.

The yoga innovator who has done the most to promote an awareness of the need to tailor a yoga practice to an individual's needs, especially taking into account the phase of life in which they are, is American yoga teacher and innovator Gary Kraftsow. A student of Desikachar, Kraftsow founded the American Viniyoga Institute (AVI), through which he educates the public about the principles of his Viniyoga (see "Viniyoga," page 107).

As Kraftsow notes, for children and teens, yoga can support balanced growth and development. For men entering and proceeding through adulthood, yoga can help promote vibrant health and support productivity and creativity. For more mature men, yoga can help promote health and well-being while fostering the quest for deeper spiritual meaning, which often accompanies this stage in a man's life. The many ways in which yoga can support you in various phases of your life journey are included in the following sections.[3]

Yoga for Boys and Teens

You don't have to be a grown man to practice yoga. Boys and teens can be especially graceful and adept yogis because of their natural flexibility, spontaneity, and eagerness to learn. Starting boys off early on the path of yoga can be one of the greatest gifts a loving parent can offer. It starts children at an early age on a path of health and wellness, while encouraging the development of strength, endurance, suppleness, grace, and balance.

In fact, many common yoga sequences were developed for young boys. Yoga colleges, or schools, for boys were established in India in the late 19th and early 20th centuries to offer young boys a full education, including physical culture. These schools were originally reserved exclusively for male students. Today, children throughout the world can practice yoga to support the balanced growth of body and mind.

Many of the flowing styles of yoga were specifically developed to meet the needs of growing and active boys—combining a sense of movement and gymnastics with the execution of the classical yoga asanas. Yoga for children can be filled with the joy of movement and spontaneous self-discovery. The weight-bearing postures of yoga can help develop strong bones, while bending and twisting movements can help ensure flexibility. A regular practice of yoga can help children to become more centered and learn at an early age to deal more effectively with stress. The yogic practices of concentration and sound breathing are gifts that can help guide a child throughout his entire life journey.

Stress is endemic today—not only among adult men. Yoga's ability to help calm and center is proving to have an increasing benefit for children. A growing number of elementary and high schools are introducing yoga practices into their curriculum in order to help students learn at an early age how to manage stress.[4] In a particularly innovative program, Krishna Kaur, a teacher and practitioner of kundalini yoga (see Chapter 7) has developed a nonprofit organization called Yoga for Youth (YFY).[5] With teachers in Chicago, Los Angeles, and New York City, Kaur and her associates teach yoga to elementary, junior, and high school students. YFY also takes yoga into the juvenile detention system—teaching the principles of a yoga lifestyle to incarcerated youngsters in an attempt to help break a cycle of attachment to criminal activities while they are still young enough to do so.

Yoga is for all children, not only troubled ones. Many yoga institutes, studios, and residential retreats offer yoga programs specifically designed for children. So, too, do many local community recreational centers. So if you would like to help a child get a head start on life, start checking out your local yoga offerings.

Yoga for Men in Their 20s and 30s

One should cultivate the highest good while the senses are not yet frail, suffering is not yet firmly rooted, and adversities have not yet become overwhelming.[6]

—*Kula-Arnava-Tantra*

Oftentimes, men come to yoga later in their lives, when they begin to experience physical problems, or reach a point where they are looking for a practice that will help them to de-stress and provide a holistic alternative to traditional physical exercise. The stresses of modern life seem to be accelerating, however, more and more for younger men, too. Overload seems to come from nearly every front—work, home, personal relations, and even the sometimes bewildering choice of leisure activities. The increasing possibilities afforded by modern conveniences and technology are leading some men to feel overwhelmed at increasingly younger ages.

Yoga can be a perfect practice for men in their 20s and 30s. In addition to empowering younger men to better manage stress, yoga can help them to maintain muscle strength and flexibility, while keeping the fullest range of motion in their joints. It can help to improve circulation, promote proper functioning of the internal organs, and help to steady the nerves. If you are in your 20s or 30s, are in good health, and wish to begin a more vigorous type of yoga practice, you might consider some of the more active approaches to yoga, such as Ashtanga Yoga, Bikram's Yoga, or Viniyoga, for instance.

Perhaps of even greater importance, yoga can help men in their 20s and 30s to lay a solid foundation for a lifetime of vibrant health. While many younger men are drawn to yoga for the physical benefits of its hatha yoga exercises, the practices of meditation and yogic breathing can lay the foundation for a smooth transition into the later phases of life. Yoga can help younger men develop healthy ways of coping with stress and caring for the body internally as well as externally—giving them a leg up on the challenges they will face throughout the rest of their lives.

Yoga can be a perfect complement to other physical exercise activities (see Chapter 12). The younger man can incorporate yoga into an all-around physical maintenance regimen, which could include not only yoga, but also other favored sports. Yoga can help to prepare a man's body for the physical demands of other activities while helping it to recover after physical activity.

Frequently, as a man begins to practice yoga, he finds that his awareness about not only his physical body, but *all* aspects of his being, becomes sharper. He begins to lead a healthier lifestyle—not because he is forcing himself to, but just because it "feels right." This subtle and spontaneous aspect of yoga is one of its best-kept secrets. If you start practicing yoga at an early age, you may well find yourself engaging in a more expanded yoga lifestyle—a lifestyle that will help guide you through the rest of your life. So if you're in your 20s and 30s, start your yoga practice as early as possible: Lay the seeds for not only a present but also a future of healthy, stress-free living. You'll be glad you did.

Yoga for Men in Their 40s and 50s

Aldous Huxley has remarked in one of his novels that the scourge of the Middle Ages was Black Death; the plague of the twentieth century is Grey Life.[7]

—Sachindra Kumar Majumdar

As men age further, the emphasis of yoga shifts again. Yoga practices can still help to protect and safeguard health, but can take on deeper spiritual dimensions. As a man matures, the emphasis of yoga practice shifts from growing strong bones, muscles, and minds in the first several decades of life to maintaining and protecting his health. It is in their 40s and 50s that men often begin to feel those nagging aches and pains that are becoming chronic. Years of strain on the body are having their toll. By their 40s and 50s, most men have established their place in the world and have reached, or are nearing, financial security. It is at this stage of life, too, that a man's attention often begins to focus less on material acquisitions and more on the examination of spiritual issues, as he takes stock of his life accomplishments and goals he has yet to achieve.

Yoga can be a perfect way to continue to maintain strength and flexibility while tailoring a routine to your particular physical needs. This can mean using yoga to help you reduce areas of pain and holding by yoga stretching techniques or continuing to maintain your body in optimal condition so that you can protect it from potential injury and strain. As men become older, it is increasingly important to protect such key areas as joints (especially at the shoulders, hips, knees, and ankles) and the muscles and vertebrae of the back. Yoga can help you to maintain strong and open joint areas as well as promote a strong and flexible back.

In addition to its physical benefits, yoga can help satisfy the emotional, mental, and psychological needs of men in their 40s and 50s. It is during these decades that men frequently begin to ask themselves with ever-greater insistence the deeper questions of life: "Who am I?", "Why am I here?", and "What is my purpose in life?" By helping you to focus and look inward, yoga can help you to explore these questions in an atmosphere of calmness, clarity, and support. Frequently, the answers to these questions will present themselves, spontaneously, in moments of silence that accompany or follow yoga practice. In this respect, it is particularly helpful if you are in your 40s and 50s to expand the yoga practices of meditation and pranayama, or breath awareness, as part of your yoga routine, or begin to incorporate them more fully if you haven't to date. You'll be glad you did, as these practices will help you weather the needs and challenges of the decades to come.

Yoga for Men in Their 60s and the Decades Beyond

Dying without knowing the meaning and purpose of life is the greatest loss.[8]

—Swami Rama

As most readers are well aware, advances in healthcare are making it possible for men to live longer lives. The average life expectancy for a male in the United States in the year 2000 was 74 according to studies by the National Center for Health Statistics at the Centers for Disease Control and Prevention.[9] However, the same agency reported that while Americans are living longer, they are not necessarily living better: They are overweight, physically lazy, and spending more money on healthcare than any other country in the world. Now, as never before, it's vital for older American men to attend to their health.

Seniors can benefit immensely from the practice of yoga. If you're in your 60s or beyond, then it's time you should seriously consider incorporating yoga into your life. If you're in your 60s or beyond and already have a regular practice of yoga, you already know the value of yoga firsthand.

For some men, yoga only begins in the senior years, when more traditional and physically demanding fitness and sports activities may place too much strain on the body. Because yoga can be practiced in an easy and gentle manner, it is ideal for individuals who may be suffering from lack of flexibility, poor range of motion, or other problems that come with older age. Yoga can help to promote flexibility and strength; increase range of motion in joints; and improve the functioning of the circulatory, immune, and endocrine systems. It can help promote enhanced functioning of the nervous system and the internal organs. It can help calm and relax, thus relieving anxiety and stress. The power of yoga to help balance and harmonize body and mind can also be an aid to such problems as despondency and insomnia, which often accompany older age.

Because there are so many approaches to yoga, if you are an older man, you should be able to find one that is right for you. If you are fit and in good shape, then you might want to try a more active type of yoga. If you are sedentary or physically challenged, yoga has ways that can help you, too.[10]

Many yoga teachers now, especially those schooled in the Iyengar approach to yoga (see Chapter 4), are adept at using a variety of props and accessories to help you attain positions you might not be able to achieve without added support. In addition, most yoga teachers can help you adapt postures to suit your particular physical condition—for instance, modifying the approach to some poses so that you can perform them against a wall for support, while seated in a chair, or even while lying on the floor.

Many of the basic postures in "A Complete Yoga Practice Session for Men" can be of great value to older men. Of particular benefit are standing poses, such as Tree Pose (Fig. YPS.5a, b, and c) and Triangle Pose (Fig. YPS.4a and b), which help to increase stability while standing. Inversions, such as the Shoulderstand (Fig. YPS.12), can also be helpful in promoting good circulation and energizing the vital organs. Forward bending postures, such as Seated Forward Bend (Fig. YPS.6), can help to lengthen tight back and leg muscles.

As men age, it is especially necessary to be aware of any possible cautions or contraindications to yoga postures. In particular, any men with glaucoma or cardiovascular difficulties, such as high blood pressure or any other history of heart problems, should avoid inverted postures, as these postures tend to increase the flow of blood. Senior men, just as men of any age, should consult with their primary healthcare provider before undertaking any new regimen of exercise.

Frequently, older age is accompanied by challenges to a man's health as well as to his outlook on life. Not only physical limitations, but also depression and anxiety can be part of older men's lives. The focusing practices of yoga can help older men gain greater clarity on their life situations—to accept themselves as they are. Often, the simple awareness and acceptance of one's limitations is a liberating experience, making many daily concerns slip by the wayside. The older man who has established a practice of meditation and pranayama in the early decades of his life will readily see how important these life tools are to him in older age, as well as younger.

For men in their senior years, the emphasis on yoga may switch from the physical aspects of the practice to meditation and breath awareness. These practices can help older men become more relaxed and centered as they delve even more deeply into the essential questions of "Who am I?" and "Why am I here?"

In India, traditions have developed that acknowledge a man's need to honor his quest for spiritual unfoldment. Some men choose to follow a time-honored custom practiced by older men: Once they have fulfilled thier "householder" duties, such as raising a family and providing financial security for their dependents, they renounce the world and leave their homes to wander the country as beggars—meditating and seeking enlightenment. A man who follows such a path might become a *sadhu* ("holy man," from the Sanskrit for "good" or "holy") or a *sannyasin* ("monk" or "ascetic," from the Sanskrit for "casting off").

You don't necessarily need to go to this extent to realize your true self. Yoga practices such as meditation and breath awareness can help to increase inner focus so that you can explore life's mysteries without ever having to leave the comfort of your own home.

The "Suggested Further Resources" section can provide you with some valuable tools to accompany you should you wish to deepen your own personal spiritual journey with yoga.

Yoga for Your "Current" Age

Yoga has the tools and resources to help every man, whatever his age. When determining what yoga practice may be right for you at your particular age, you may want to take into consideration the physical condition of your body as well as your chronological age.[11] Take stock of your own personal state of health and fitness. A man in his 20s who is in poor health or who is compromised physically may want to do a gentler yoga practice. A man in his 60s who has a vibrant body and mind may be able to do a more active yoga practice than some other men of his age. So when setting out a program of yoga for yourself, consider your biological, physical condition as well as your chronological age. Your yoga teacher should be able to help you in tailoring a yoga program to suit your particular needs— whatever your age.

Yoga for Your Physical Condition

A man can encounter physical problems at any stage in his life journey. You'll find more information on how yoga can help with specific health concerns and issues in Chapter 13.

Suggested Further Resources

Gary Kraftsow, who popularized Viniyoga, is the foremost spokesperson for how yoga can help people at different stages of their lives. To find out more about his approach to yoga, see "Viniyoga" on page 107.

You might also want to explore the following title:

Srivatsa Ramaswami, *Yoga for the Three Stages of Life: Developing Your Practice as an Art Form, a Physical Therapy, and a Guiding Philosophy* (Inner Traditions, 2000). In this book, the author, a student of legendary teacher Krishnamacharya, focuses on how to adapt yoga to individual needs and to different stages of life.

If you'd like to explore further how yoga can help you, a friend, or loved one at specific life stages, the following additional resources are recommended.

Yoga for Boys and Teens

If you'd like to help a child or teen understand that yoga can be fun and cool, these are helpful starting points:

Laurent de Brunhoff, *Babar's Yoga for Elephants* (Harry W. Abram, 2002). This book was created by the extraordinarily talented and prolific originator of the Babar series of children's books, Laurent de Brunhoff, who maintains a daily yoga practice himself. In this whimsically engaging book, Babar shares 15 yoga asanas and stretches sure to appeal to the child in your life, or to the child in you.

Jodi B. Komitor, M.A., and Eve Adamson, *Complete Idiot's Guide to Yoga with Kids* (Alpha Books Press, 2000). Using the simple and fun style of the *Complete Idiot* series of offerings, this book will help you introduce your children to yoga, whether or not you're a guru.

Lisa Trivell, *I Can't Believe It's Yoga for Kids* (Heatherleigh Press, 2000). Written by a certified yoga instructor and fitness professional with experience teaching yoga in public and private schools, this book features kids performing yoga in a cool way that may help inspire the children who are important in your life.

Children are often more inspired by the immediate visual impact of films than books. The following videos present yoga to kids in a fun and playful way:

E-i-E-i Yoga for Kids (Mystic Fire Video, 1996). This video, which takes place in a barnyard setting, features mature yogi Max Thomas introducing a group of children to a simple yet complete yoga practice. Thomas's display of gymnastics and acrobatics as he presents the routine may be just the thing to inspire your child at an early age to pursue yoga as a lifelong journey.

Gaiam/Living Arts presents a series of fun 30-minute videos for children. *Yoga for Kids* is geared to children ages 3 to 6. *Yoga Fitness for Kids* is available in one version as a video for children ages 3 to 6, and in another version for children ages 7 to 12 (Gaiam/Living Arts, 1996 and 2001, respectively).

Yoga for Men in Their 20s and 30s

If you're in your 20s or 30s, you may be interested in practicing a more vigorous approach to yoga. If what you're looking for is a sweaty program that makes your heart as well as the rest of your body work hard, you may be interested in exploring Ashtanga, or Power, Yoga. Chapter 6 includes resources for further information on Ashtanga Yoga.

As yoga is catching on with younger males, books featuring fit and active young male presenters of yoga are now available. You may be interested in checking out one of these offerings:

Baron Baptiste, *Journey into Power: How to Sculpt Your Ideal Body, Free Your True Self, and Transform Your Life with Yoga* (Fireside, 2002). Celebrated for his "Journey into Power" yoga boot camps with yoga postures performed in heated rooms, this book integrates the principles of Baptiste's vigorous physical yoga exercises with the spiritual dimensions of yoga practice.

Rodney Yee, *Yoga: The Poetry of the Body* (St. Martin's Press, 2002). This is a handsomely produced book, presenting one of the most well-known male yoga teachers.

Yoga for Men in Their 40s and 50s

If you're in your 40s or 50s, you may be interested in taking your yoga practice to a new level by becoming even more precise in your practice and learning ways in which you can adapt your yoga practice to your particular physical condition and needs. Iyengar Yoga offers a particularly precise approach to yoga, including ways in which you can use props to modify poses for your particular needs, as well as helping prescribe practice programs for varying physical limitations. For more information, see the resources included in Chapter 4.

As you advance on life's journey, you may also feel that you are looking for a less vigorous, more relaxed, yet still energizing approach to yoga. The Himalayan Institute (Chapter 2),

Integral Yoga (Chapter 3), and Sivananda Yoga (Chapter 5) may be right for you—you'll find suggested resources for each of these approaches to yoga in their respective chapters.

In your 40s and 50s, you may also be interested in incorporating the yogic principles of meditation and pranayama, or yogic breathing, more fully into your yoga practice. If so, see the suggested resources on these practices in Chapter 16.

If you're entering your more mature years, you may find the following book custom-tailored to where you are in the stream of life:

Suza Francina, *The New Yoga for People over 50: A Comprehensive Guide for Midlife and Older Beginners* (Health Communications, 1997). This is an excellent introduction to yoga for mature men. Written by a yoga teacher trained in Iyengar Yoga, it presents a comprehensive overview of yoga for the older practitioner—whether one just starting out or a veteran yogi. It contains ample information on how to modify poses through the use of props, some as simple as chairs and walls, so that virtually anyone can achieve the benefits of yoga.

Yoga for Men in Their 60s and Beyond

If you're in your 60s or beyond, you may be interested in easy approaches to yoga that help keep the joints mobile and the circulation steady. The following book contains a series of joint and gland exercises that are easy to perform:

Rudolph Ballentine, M.D., editor, *Joints and Glands Exercises: As Taught by Sri Swami Rama of the Himalayas* (Himalayan Institute Press, 1977). This is an excellent overview of a series of easy-to-perform yoga exercises that can be particularly helpful to seniors.

As you progress in your senior years, you may find that your interest in the spiritual aspects of yoga deepens even more. The following books on the spiritual foundations of yoga might be of particular interest:

Bernard Bouanchaud (Rosemary Desneux, trans.) *The Essence of Yoga: Reflections on the Yoga Sutras of Patanjali*. (Rudra Press, 1997). This book uses the time-honored tradition of teaching the foundational principles of yoga by presenting in translation and then commenting upon the terse aphorisms of the first recorded expert on yoga, Patanjali.

Swami Venkatesananda, *The Concise Yoga Vasistha* (State University of New York, 1985). This is a highly readable abridgement of one of the greatest and most profound scriptures of yogic philosophy.

Many yoga experts consider the *Bhagavad Gita* to be the "bible" of yoga philosophy. There are many translations and commentaries available upon this seminal yogic text, which forms an essential part of the most sacred yogic writings, the *Upanishads*. If you're interested in going right to the source, visit your local library or bookstore and select the version of the *Bhagavad Gita* that appeals most to your inner knowing.

One of the most accomplished practitioners and teachers of the yoga of self-discovery in the 20th century was Jean Klein (1916–1998.) A musicologist and medical doctor from Central Europe, Klein pursued a lifetime practice of Advaita Vedanta, a branch of yogic philosophy concerned with inquiry into the self. He taught his students an approach to exploring the mind and self-awareness, both in Europe and in the United States. His teachings are available in a series of books, with such apt titles as *Who Am I?, Be Who You Are,* and

I Am. You can find out more about Jean Klein and his work by visiting the Website of the Jean Klein Foundation at *www.jeanklein.org.*

Richard Miller studied with both T.K.V. Desikachar and Jean Klein. His Website contains information and links to other sites that explore inquiry into the self: *www.nondual.com.*

Finally, as you enter your senior years, don't forget that among the major paths of yoga is that of karma yoga, the yoga of liberation through devotion and service to something greater than yourself. If you're in your 60s or beyond and have some time to share, consider volunteering for a worthy organization: In this way, you can put your lifetime of experience to good use in a conscious and active approach to yoga practice that will help to serve the planet while making you feel good as well.

Gary Kraftsow on yoga for the phases of a man's life:

"As children, our practice should support the balanced growth and development of body and mind. As adults, our practice should protect health and promote the ability to be productive in the world. As seniors, our practice should help us maintain health and inspire the deeper quest for self-realization."[12]

—Gary Kraftsow, Founder of the American Viniyoga Institute

Chapter 12

YOGA FOR ATHLETICS AND SPORTS

How to Use Yoga to Make the Most of Your Fitness Activities

I believe that my achievements as a coach/psychologist are 60 to 70 percent due to my coaching ability, and 30 to 40 percent due to yoga preparation and self-regulation.[1]

—Aladar Kogler, Ph.D., Olympic Fencing Coach and Director of the Columbia University Sports Psychology Research Laboratory

"Is yoga for real men?" you might be asking yourself if you're new to yoga.

"Yes, it is!" is the resounding answer to this question, which is sometimes raised by men who may be new to yoga. An underlying tenet of *Yoga for Men* is that yoga is for every man—athletes included. In this chapter, you'll find out how yoga can help enhance your ongoing athletic and sports activities in addition to providing a complete program itself for maintaining and improving strength of body, mind, and soul.

Yoga and You: Challenges Confronting the "Macho" Man

If you're already practicing yoga or are being drawn to yoga out of a driving fascination, then you don't need to be convinced that it is for you. But if you're like a lot of men, especially of the "macho" variety or a guy who's addicted to weightlifting or vigorous athletic sport, you may be a bit skeptical or even apprehensive about approaching a practice of yoga. You may feel that it's a practice for women, wimps, or spiritual escapists. Or you may feel a different kind of apprehension—a fear that you won't be able to do yoga postures as well as other men who have been practicing for a long time, or will be viewed with contempt as a yoga "outsider."[2]

While such fears are natural, they shouldn't keep you from pursuing yoga. It is true that in recent Western history, yoga has been practiced more by women than by men. However, throughout the history of yoga, many of its practices, particularly the physical postures of hatha yoga, were reserved exclusively for male practitioners. An increasing number of men today are discovering and embracing the vibrant power that yoga has offered men for thousands of years. And frequently to their surprise, they are finding that yoga can provide a complete workout for body, mind, and spirit that can enhance their performance in other physical activities and even replace or spice up that boring old gym workout. Indeed, no less an icon of virility than Richard Gere, once named "Sexiest Man of the Year" by *Time*, has reportedly traded in the workout bench for a yoga mat.[3]

You don't have to go to the extreme of giving up your everyday athletic activities to benefit from the strengthening, toning, and centering benefits of yoga, though. Many professional athletes find yoga a powerful way to enhance their own physical performance: The Florida Marlins benefited from a yoga coach during their 1997 season, when they won the World Series.[4] Many other accomplished athletes swear by yoga, as well. In the following sections, you'll find just some of the ways in which yoga can help enhance your ongoing athletic and fitness activities.

How Yoga Can Help You Make the Most of Your Fitness Activities

Many men come to the practice of yoga through the "back door": Avid athletes who injure themselves turn to yoga as a last resort alternative to mend and restore their bodies. While yoga can help you to recover from a sports injury, you don't have to do yourself bodily injury before you can benefit from it. In fact, yoga is one of the best fitness activities to help prevent injury from occurring in the first place. Yoga practices can help you enhance your performance in nearly any physical activity by preparing you for the activity beforehand, guiding you with mindful awareness through its performance and helping to restore you afterward. In addition, it can help you strengthen yourself further by helping you to compensate for areas of your body that are not exercised by your sport so as to have full and complete overall body strength and vitality.

Yoga can help you to prepare to engage in your fitness activity or sport by strengthening, stretching, and toning your overall musculature. Practicing a basic yoga session (for example, "A Complete Yoga Practice Session for Men" on page 112) can help improve the functioning and tone of all the muscles of your body, as well as increase flexibility and range of motion in joints, improve circulation, and promote optimal functioning of your internal organs. Thus, you'll be better prepared to practice your sport with much less risk of injury, as you benefit from enhanced muscular and joint strength and flexibility, and perhaps even improved breathing capacity.

Once you practice your sport, yoga can help you to stay present and aware during your activity. With increased attention, you're bound to perform better. You'll be more aware of your movements and be better able to remember—and learn from—any shortcomings in your performance. The balancing postures of yoga—such as Tree Pose (Fig. YPS.5a, b, and c, page 124)—are especially beneficial for developing a sense of centeredness and balance that will serve you well in the execution of any sport. Should you opt to incorporate the practice of meditation into your yoga practice, you may be pleasantly surprised to discover your sense of balance and grace growing even further as you reach an athlete's "high," wherein you attain that blissful state of "meditation in motion" while you enjoy your favorite fitness activity.

Once you've finished your sports activity, yoga stretching can help in the elimination of toxic waste substances that your body builds up during exercise, as well as lengthen and restore muscles to their relaxed state following peak exertion. This can help in any sport, including weightlifting. In fact, studies have shown that muscles that are stretched are able to lift more weight and actually become stronger as the result of the stretching.[5] Doing yoga stretching after physical exercise can also be very helpful because your muscles and other body tissues are already warmed up by your physical activity. This means that you'll be able to stretch further than you could if your muscles were "cold." When stretching after physical exertion, be especially mindful to move slowly into your stretch and to hold it at its maximum point for at least 20 to 30 seconds if you can. And, as with any stretching, don't bounce or jerk yourself into position. Move slowly, gradually, and mindfully, allowing your breath to take you to your deepest stretch. Never stretch to the point of pain or beyond your level of comfort. Respect your body and yourself.

Finally, incorporating yoga into your fitness practice may actually help you achieve a level of overall physical conditioning that is more complete and more balanced than that which you may be achieving by practicing your particular athletic activity on its own. Most sports activities tend to use certain body parts or one side of the body rather than all parts of the body equally. For instance, a runner may emphasize the use of the legs and feet; a boxer, the hands, arms, and upper body; and a tennis player uses one arm, hand, and shoulder more than the other. Such tendencies can result in imbalances in the strength and tone of your musculature, which, in turn, can translate into postural imbalances. Overuse of certain muscle groups or joints can also lead to pain and an increased chance of injury. By being aware of how you are using your body, you can consciously tailor a yoga program to fit your specific fitness needs while simultaneously stretching and toning all the major muscle groups of your body.

Tailoring a Yoga Program to Your Specific Fitness and Sports Needs

You can easily custom-tailor a yoga program to meet your specific needs. As an overall recommendation, be sure to include stretching before and after your physical activity. Try to include stretches that address the entire body. You can choose from among the yoga exercises provided in "A Complete Yoga Practice Session for Men." For instance, performing a round of Sun Salutations will provide a stretch for the entire body. You could also choose a complete stretching program by choosing to perform one yoga exercise from each of the major categories of yoga postures—for instance, you could choose one forward bending exercise from among Standing Forward Bend (Fig. YPS.1d, page 116), Seated Forward Bend

(Fig. YPS.6, page 125), or Head-to-Knee Pose (Fig. YPS.7, page 126); one backward bend-ing exercise from among Cobra Pose (Fig. YPS.8, page 127), Bow Pose (Fig. YPS.9, page 129), or Bridge Pose (Fig. YPS.11, page 131); one twisting exercise, such as Seated Spinal Twist (Fig. YPS.10, page 124); and one inversion, such as Downward-Facing Dog (Fig. YPS.1j, page 118) or Shoulderstand (Fig. YPS.12, page 132). To provide as varied a pro-gram as possible, try alternating the poses you choose. For instance, if you choose to do Cobra Pose as your backbend exercise one day, try to do Bridge or Bow Pose as an alternative the next time you work out.

To hone in more precisely on your particular sport, you might also want to choose some yoga exercises that help to stretch and strengthen certain body parts—in particular, the ones that relate most specifically to your particular sport. For example, for tennis you might want to choose yoga postures such as Triangle Pose (Fig. YPS.4a and b, page 123) and Eagle Pose (Fig. 14.2, page 186) that help to open and rotate the arm and shoulder. For running, you may want to choose poses that help to strengthen and tone the legs, such as Tree Pose (Fig. YPS5a, b, and c, page 124); or relax the hamstrings, such as Standing Forward Bend (Fig. YPS.1d, page 116) or Seated Forward Bend (Fig. YPS.6, page 125). For rowing, you might want to choose poses that help strengthen and stretch the back, such as Bow Pose (Fig. YPS.9, page 129). You can also incorporate poses that help work body parts that are neglected in your particular sports activity. For instance, if you're a hiker, you might want to do some poses that emphasize the arms, shoulders, and upper body, such as Bridge Pose (Fig. YPS.11, page 131), or Shoulderstand (Fig. YPS.12, page 122).

It's important to help your body to integrate the benefits that you're achieving by your physical activity and to heal and restore itself. So be sure to include some restorative yoga poses in your program. Corpse Pose (Fig. YPS.3, page 122) and Legs-up-the Wall Pose (Fig. 13.3, page 164) are examples of excellent restorative postures.

Finally, yoga can help you perform and recover from your athletic fitness activities with more than just its collection of asanas, or physical exercise postures. Proper diet, breathing exercises, and a meditation practice can all help you go that extra distance in your chosen activity. To begin to incorporate the full range of yoga tools into your fitness and wellness practice, see Chapter 16, which discusses the yoga lifestyle.

Suggested Further Resources

In this chapter, you've seen how you can incorporate yoga into your fitness program and devise a blueprint for a custom-tailored yoga program. Each particular sport and fit-ness activity can have its own unique yoga plan. If you'd like more information on specific postures and stretches that you can explore for your specific fitness activities and goals, the following resources are highly recommended to supplement the information presented in this chapter.

Books

Aladar Kogler, Ph.D., is the foremost expert on how you can use yoga to help enhance your athletic performance. The guidance presented in his book provided much of the back-ground information in this chapter. His book is highly recommended:

Aladar Kogler, Ph.D., *Yoga for Athletes: Secrets of an Olympic Coach* (Llewellyn, 1999). This is a comprehensive reference book on how you can incorporate yoga into your particular sports or fitness activity. The author, a fencing coach at Columbia University and director of the Columbia University Sports Psychology Research Laboratory, draws on his years of experience in incorporating yoga into the fitness training programs of high-level, Olympic champion athletes to show how every man can benefit from yoga. He explains in detail how yoga can help improve performance in various athletic activities, as well as how specific yoga postures can help compensate for the overuse of certain muscle groups in specific sports.

Bob Anderson's book on stretching is the classic introduction to stretching for every sports activity. While not specifically presenting yoga postures, many of the stretches he suggests in his book mirror classical yoga postures:

Bob Anderson, *Stretching: 20th Anniversary Revised Edition* (Shelter Publications, 2000). This is a sound basic manual on stretching that has been translated into 16 languages with millions of copies sold around the world. The author does an excellent job of introducing the theory behind stretching and detailing how you can develop a complete stretching program to accompany your particular athletic activity. Stretching routines are provided for more than 20 sports-specific activities, including such popular categories as running, tennis, racquetball, cycling, swimming, golf, weight training, and more.

Video

Bob Anderson, *Stretching: The Video* (Shelter Publications, 1987). This is the videotape companion to the classic text on stretching cited previously.

Yoga Conditioning for Athletes with Rodney Yee (Gaiam/Living Arts, 2000). Featuring yoga superstar Rodney Yee, this 60-minute video is designed to help you improve your athletic ability and play longer with fewer injuries, no matter what your sport.

Body Wisdom Media has produced an innovative, interactive DVD that can help you tailor a yoga program to your specific athletic needs:

Yoga for Athletes Interactive Yoga Series (Body Wisdom Media, 2002). This interactive DVD responds to each athlete's specific needs by offering 12 customized workouts for 16 different sports. Routines range from 20 to 60 minutes. Sports presented include cycling, golf, hiking, skiing, swimming, tennis, volleyball, weightlifting, and more.

Website

The following Website contains links to articles on stretching archived in its stretch library of articles: *www.yoga.com.*

Vince Serecin on yoga for men:

"The men that come to my yoga classes are often the most resistant. Many times, their trainers send them to my class to help them become more flexible. Yoga is one of the best all-around workouts because it can help men build strength and at the same time become more flexible. It can help men relieve stiff backs and sore muscles, while reducing stress and boosting energy levels.

"I work on Wall Street, not far from the World Trade Center. Many men come to me with concerns about stress and how to eliminate it through yoga. I have often fielded questions about chronic pain, sports injuries, problems after surgery, or repetitive stress injuries. Yoga can help all of these issues. Yoga is the panacea of all ills—not only in the body, but also in the mind."

—Vince Serecin, Yoga Instructor at New York Sports Clubs in Manhattan

Jimmy Barkan on yoga and baseball:

"Practicing yoga, when you have to stay within yourself and in the moment, helps in the field."[6]

—Jimmy Barkan, Owner of the Yoga College of India in
Fort Lauderdale, Florida

Guy Mezger on yoga and kickboxing:

"The second your mind wanders is the second your opponent moves in."[7]

—Guy Mezger, Owner of Freestyle Martial Arts in Dallas and Author of
The Complete Idiot's Guide to Kickboxing

Chapter 13

YOGA FOR MEN'S HEALTH

How Yoga Can Help You Maintain Your Health/Address Specific Men's Health Concerns

...The body is a wonderful instrument.... You should take care of it properly. An unhealthy body dissipates the mind—you then have no time to work with other aspects of yourself. That is why maintaining physical health is an integral part of spiritual practice.[1]

—Swami Rama

Yoga is one of the best overall integrated healthcare systems available. In India, yoga practices form an integral part of the healing methods of *ayurveda* (the "science of life" or "science of health" in Sanskrit). Ayurvedic medicine is a 5,000-year-old system of healing based on the sacred Vedic literature of India. It is the oldest continuously practiced system of healthcare in the world. Ayurvedic medicine utilizes a variety of means to promote health and well-being, including herbs, crystals, aromatic essences and oils, massage, and, most importantly, the use of principles and practices drawn from the yoga tradition.

In India, the practice of yoga has, until recently, been the nearly exclusive domain of men. Virtually all the Indian masters who brought the teachings of yoga to the West were men, as seen in Part II of this book. Ironically, however, yoga in the West has been practiced largely by women, depriving today's man of yoga's many valuable health benefits. The goal of *Yoga for Men* is to help make yoga a part of every man's program for overall fitness and healthy living.

In a very general sense, the practice of yoga is an excellent way for virtually every single man to maintain his health. Yoga postures promote strength, flexibility, good circulation, increased range of motion in joints, and optimal functioning of the internal organs. A yogic diet promotes the proper nutrition that your body needs for growth and repair. Yogic breathing exercises help to remove waste products resulting from your body's metabolic processes, while providing fresh oxygen for renewed vigor and energy. Meditation can help you calm your mind's chatter to contact your deepest sources of well-being, helping you to reduce and better mange stress while making your mind even clearer and more creative. Yoga can also help every man to open his heart more fully to the beauty and joy that the universe has in store for everyone.

The best time to start practicing yoga is now—whatever your age or physical condition. If you are healthy, the regular and disciplined practice of yoga can help you to maintain your health and fortify your body to ward off potential illness more effectively. If you suffer from a particular health concern, yoga may help you alleviate the condition. And through the mindfulness that a sustained yoga practice engenders, chances are that you'll be much more in touch and aware of your body so as to take appropriate measures to attend to any potential health problems.

Following are just some of the ways in which yoga can address a number of the most common health issues of concern to men.

Yoga and Your Back

One of the most common health problems afflicting men is a "bad back." You may have already had the experience of back pain. And chances are that if you haven't, you will: It is estimated that 80 percent of adult Americans suffer from back pain at some point during their lives.[2] Back pain is the most frequent cause of employee lost work time—more than any other occupational disorder.[3] And the chief complaint among men who suffer from back pain is pain in the lower back.

While some back pain is caused by accidents or genetics, much back pain is caused by faulty posture, and so it is avoidable. Yoga is a great way for you to help improve the state of your back. In fact, one of the principal goals of yoga is to promote a strong, healthy, and flexible spine so that the dormant kundalini energy that lies coiled like a serpent at the base of the spine can rise in a smooth and unimpeded flow up the central energy channel of the sushumna that lies in the center of the spinal column (see Chapter 7).

The most common source of back pain is weak or tight muscles in the back, abdomens, and hamstrings. Back problems are often exacerbated by today's man's sedentary lifestyle, which not only causes strain in the lower back, but also often leads to obesity. Yoga exercises that address the muscles of the abdomen, back, and hamstrings along with the principles of a yogic diet are boons to any man concerned with the health of his back.

Frequently, the muscles of the back and hamstrings are tight, while those of the abdomen are weak. This puts strain all along the entire back and spine, and particularly at the area of the lower back. Yoga exercises that strengthen and stretch the muscles of the back and abdomen can do a lot to help relieve back pain.

Specific yoga postures that can help you care for your back include all of the backward and forward bends presented in "A Complete Yoga Practice Session for Men." Generally, backward bends help to strengthen the muscles of the back and hamstrings, while forward bends help to stretch and release them. Some forward bends can also help relieve compression on the sciatic nerve, which can be a source of pain. Backward bends presented in a "A Complete Yoga Practice Session for Men" include Cobra Pose (Fig. YPS.8, page 127), Bow Pose (Fig. YPS.9, page 129), and Bridge Pose (Fig. YPS.11, page 131). Forward bends include Standing Forward Bend (Fig. YPS.1d, page 116), Child's Pose (Fig. YPS.2a and b, page 121), Seated Forward Bend (Fig. YPS.6, page 125), and Head-to-Knee Pose (Fig. YPS.7, page 126). Try doing these postures to strengthen and stretch the muscles of your back. In addition, you can practice Seated Spinal Twist (Fig. YPS.10, page 129) to strengthen and increase the flexibility of the entire lower back and abdominal area.

Because the back is such an important, and problematic, area for many men, the following are several additional yoga exercises and modifications that you may find helpful in attending to the care of your back. You can do these yoga asanas any time and anywhere you like as independent, stress-busting poses. You can also try incorporating them into your practice of "A Complete Yoga Practice Session for Men" for added variety.

Uttanasana: Standing Forward Bend

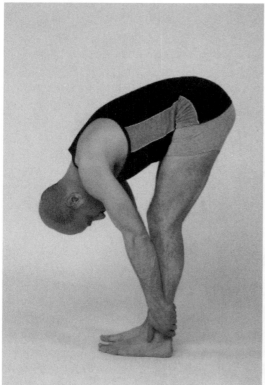 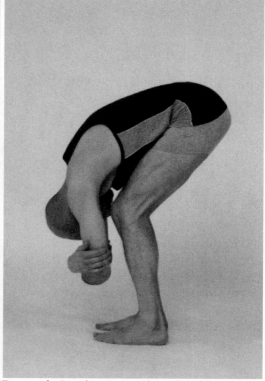

Fig. 13.1a: Standing Forward Bend With Knees Bent, Grasping the Ankle

Fig. 13.1b: Standing Forward Bend Holding Elbows While Dangling

Uttanasana, or "Standing Forward Bend," is introduced as Position 3 in the Sun Salutation series (Fig. YPS.1d, page 116), where it is described and illustrated in the full pose. This asana is a great stress-buster for relieving both physical and mental tension.

It's possible to practice modified variations of Standing Forward Bend for a gentler and more restorative approach to releasing tension in the back and hamstring muscles. In the full pose, the upper torso is folded over the legs. The legs remain as straight as possible and the palms of the hands are placed alongside the feet, fingertips in line with the toes (see Fig. YPS.1d, page 116).

One variation of Standing Forward Bend is to fold the upper torso forward while you keep the knees bent, and grasp the ankles or shins with your hands to help give you support (see Fig. 13.1a). Another variation is to rest your torso over your thighs as you hold each elbow with the hand of the opposite arm (see Fig. 13.1b).

These modified approaches to Standing Forward Bend are especially easy to perform and you can do them virtually anywhere, anytime. Try practicing these poses as a "yoga break" at the office or when you get home from work as a stress-busting transition to the rest of your day.

Bidalasana: Cat Pose

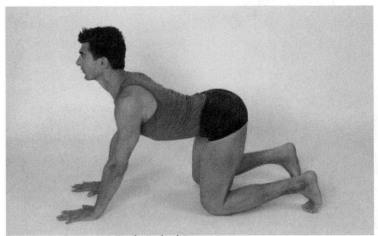

Fig. 13.2a: Cat Pose—Back Arched Down

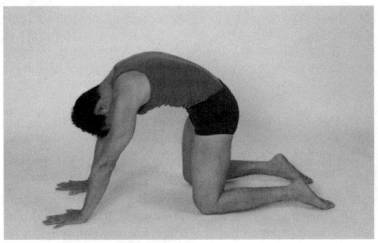

Fig. 13.2b: Cat Pose—Back Arched Up

Bidalasana (*bidala* means "cat" in Sanskrit) is most popularly referred to as "Cat Pose" or "Cat Stretch," and alternatively by some practitioners as "Cat-Cow Stretch." This stretch uses deceptively simple yoga movements that can help you strengthen and stretch the spine simultaneously.

To prepare for Cat Pose, assume a kneeling position on the floor. Try to practice this exercise on a carpeted surface or with some padding under your knees to protect them. You should be on all fours—the knees directly under the hips and the hands under the shoulders. The feet should be flexed (toes curled under) and the palms and fingers pressed firmly into the floor.

As you inhale, curve the area of your lower back downward as you lift the head, creating a hollow downward curve in the area just above the upper ridge of the back of the pelvis. Continue to inhale as you progressively increase the downward arch of the spine and back. Feel the movement extend all the way into the middle back, upper back, shoulders, neck, and head so that your nose is pointing directly forward or up. Allow your back and shoulder areas to remain wide and broad, as illustrated in Fig. 13.2a. (This is the "Cow" portion of "Cat-Cow Stretch.")

Smoothly, without pause, exhale as you reverse the curvature of your spine, once again initiating the movement in the lower back. Point your toes so that the top surfaces of the feet rest on the ground. Compress the abdominal area to initiate an exaggerated arch upward, continuing the movement through to the middle back, upper back, shoulders and, last of all, the neck and head. Your nose will now be pointing in the direction of the floor, as illustrated in Fig. 13.2b. (This is the "Cat" portion of "Cat-Cow Stretch.")

Continue to practice Cat Pose. Breathe rhythmically: as you inhale, arch your back downward; as you exhale, arch your back upward. Perform this Cat Stretch for several rounds of rhythmic breathing if you are a beginner, or for up to for several minutes if you are more experienced in the pose. As you alternately arch and round the spine, become aware of the effect of this stretch on your entire back, not just on the area around the center of the back surrounding the spine. Feel the effect of the strengthening and stretching radiating all the way out from the spine to your sides and even around to the front of the chest. As you perform these stretching movements, be aware of the movements of a cat as it spontaneously stretches its back. When you've finished performing Cat Pose, relax for a moment in Child's Pose. Be aware of how this stretch has affected you. Does your back feel differently than before you began the stretch? Do you feel differently—emotionally, mentally, and/or psychologically—as a result of this yoga posture?

Viparita Karani: Legs-up-the-Wall Pose

Viparita karani, or "Legs-up-the-Wall Pose" (*viparita* means "inverted" and *karani* means "doing") is a powerfully restorative posture. It is a variation of the Shoulderstand. In fact, this pose can be an alternative inverted posture for those men who find the Shoulderstand too challenging. Legs-up-the-Wall Pose helps to relieve backache while providing the stimulating benefits of an inverted posture, helping to promote good circulation, particularly in the legs and feet. In addition to being practiced as part of a complete yoga workout, yoga postures can be practiced individually for their specific benefits whenever and wherever you have the time and inclination to do them: Try this posture when you come home from work and want to relax and renew yourself after a stressful day. Follow the example set by the model in Fig. 13.3: take off your shoes, loosen your belt, and invert your legs up the wall.

In viparita karani, you'll be lying on the floor on your back with your legs supported above you on the wall. You may wish to have a pillow or other padded prop handy to support your lower back and hips in this position. First, find a comfortable, padded space on the floor next to a wall where you'll be able to place your legs. Sit sideways against the wall with your right side facing the wall, about five to six inches away from it. As you exhale, swivel your buttocks toward the wall as you simultaneously lift your legs straight against the wall and lower your upper body so that your back is on the floor. Check to see how this placement of your body against the wall feels. If you are stiff, or tall, you may need to slide your buttocks slightly farther from the wall. You can also try placing a pillow or other padded prop under your buttocks for additional support. Experiment until you find a comfortable position. Don't be discouraged if it seems difficult to get into position on the first few tries. You are using your body in a new way, and it can take

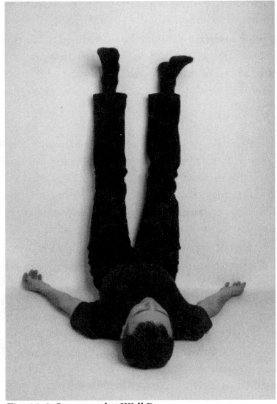

Fig. 13.3: Legs-up-the-Wall Pose

time to develop the kinesthetic sense to do the pose comfortably. This pose is deeply restorative and is well worth the effort to experiment with it. Stay in this position for a few minutes to begin and gradually increase your time in the position for up to 15 to 20 minutes. As you perform Legs-up-the-Wall Pose, allow your sternum to lift toward your chin. Avoid any strain on the neck.

Back pain can be caused by problems with the muscles of the back, and also (and commonly) as a result of weak abdominal muscles. Healthy buttocks muscles are also important to good posture, a healthy back, and an attractive appearance. The following section will help you learn how you can help build strong abdominal muscles while helping to relieve back pain at the same time. Some of these exercises will also help firm and strengthen the buttocks.

Yoga and Your Abs and Butt

Many men yearn for strong abdominal muscles because of the attractive, masculine appearance well-toned abdominal muscles help create and project. But having strong abdominal muscles has benefits much deeper than appearance. In Asian thought, the abdomen is a man's storehouse of power and energy. Having firm, yet flexible, abdominal muscles helps us maintain our sense of centeredness and power in the world. And as previously stated, strong abs can also help protect a man's back from injury and pain.

Here are some yoga exercises that you can do to help maintain the strength and health of your abdominal muscles.

Seated Cat Stretch

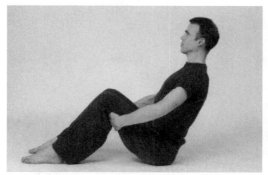 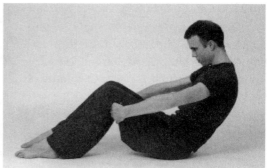

Fig. 13.4a: Seated Cat Stretch—Flat Back   Fig. 13.4b: Seated Cat Stretch—Rounded Back

In Seated Cat Stretch, you alternately strengthen and stretch your abdominal muscles. To perform this yoga posture, sit on the floor on a comfortable, padded surface with your legs bent and the soles of your feet planted on the floor in front of you. The legs are bent at the knees and the legs form an upside-down V relative to the floor. Your feet should be a comfortable distance in front of the buttocks, parallel to one another and slightly wider apart than the hips.

Place each hand on the back surface of the corresponding thigh just above the knee crease. As you inhale, expand and open your chest as you flatten and arch the back forward to bring the upper body close toward the thighs—your abdomen fills up with air (see Fig. 13.4a).

As you exhale, contract the abdominal muscles as you round the upper body backward. Compress the abdominal muscles and navel area, in particular, back in toward the spine (see Fig. 13.4b).

Inhale and arch forward again. Exhale and round your back. Continue this Seated Cat Stretch for several rounds of natural, rhythmic breathing. As you exhale, feel how your abdominal muscles are being flattened, compressed, and firmed. As you inhale, feel how they are being stretched and your lower back is being strengthened.

Standing Abdominal Lift

Standing Abdominal Lift is an abdominal squeezing exercise that you can perform while standing. It helps to strengthen the abdominal muscles while giving a powerful massage to the internal organs.

Stand in Mountain Pose (Fig. YPS.1a, page 115) with your feet firmly planted on the ground about hip-width apart, and your arms and hands by your sides. Lower the buttocks to come into a modified squat position. Place your hands on your thighs for support. As you exhale, squeeze in your abdomen as the belly lifts up, creating a hollow arch. With this exhalation, actively compress your abdominal muscles. Feel the strong contraction in the entire area of your solar plexus. Relax the abdominal muscles as you inhale fully and completely.

Once again, exhale strongly as you squeeze in your abdomen. Inhale fully and naturally and relax the abdominal muscles. Practice this posture for several rounds of full, deep, rhythmic breathing.

Navasana: Boat Pose

Navasana (literally "Boat Pose" in Sanskrit) is a very powerful pose for gaining abdominal strength, as well as for developing balance and poise. The following are directions for practicing Boat Pose in two variations: Full Boat Pose and Modified Boat Pose. Try to do Full Boat Pose. If this pose is too challenging for you, then try Modified Boat Pose. As you develop strength and stamina, continue on to Full Boat Pose.

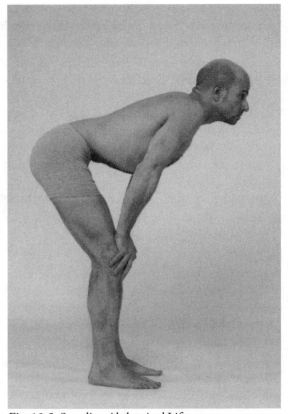

Fig. 13.5: Standing Abdominal Lift

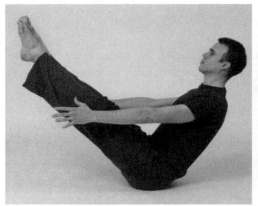

Fig. 13.6a: Full Boat Pose

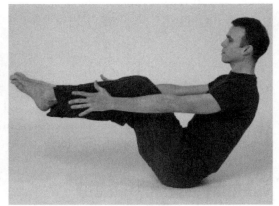

Fig. 13.6b: Modified Boat Pose

To perform Full Boat Pose (*paripurna navasana—paripurna* means "full"), begin by sitting on the floor on a comfortable padded surface with your legs bent and the soles of your feet planted on the floor in front of you, as in Seated Cat Stretch. Exhale and lift your legs off the ground. Extend them out straight in front of you and lift them as high as you can, pointing the toes. Extend your lower legs as you straighten them from the knees and point your toes up toward the ceiling. Extend your arms and hands straight out in front of you so that they are parallel to the floor. Balance as fully and securely as possible on your sit-bones and see if you can form a V, with your sit-bones forming the bottom fulcrum point of the V (see Fig. 13.6a). Breathe naturally and rhythmically for several rounds. When you are ready to release from the pose, lower your legs and your back to the ground.

If Full Boat Pose is too challenging for you or you would simply like to vary your practice, try Modified Boat Pose. Sit on a comfortable padded surface on the floor. Your legs are bent and the soles of your feet are planted flat on the ground in front of you as in preparation for Full Boat Pose. Exhale and lift your legs off the ground. Your legs remain bent at the knees as you do so. Extend your legs so that the lower legs (shins and calves) are parallel to the ground. The tips of your toes should be at about the level of your sternum. Raise your arms and hands straight in front of you, parallel to the ground and outside of your legs (see Fig. 13.6b). Hold this pose as you breathe naturally for several rounds. When you are ready to release from this pose, lower your legs to the ground.

Poses for Increasing Abdominal Awareness and Strengthening the Buttocks

Many men desire to have not only strong, attractive abs, but a well-toned butt as well! Doing an exercise that involves a pelvic lift is an excellent way for a man to increase awareness of the abdominal area while also strengthening and toning the buttocks. One of the best abdominal lifts in yoga is Bridge Pose. This asana combines a powerful pelvic lift with a back bending movement. Bridge Pose is presented in "A Complete Yoga Practice Session for Men," where it is illustrated in Fig. YPS.11 (page 131).

In addition to Bridge Pose, Locust Pose is an excellent yoga exercise to help a man increase abdominal awareness, stimulate the internal organs, and firm and tone the buttocks, while strengthening the back—all at the same time!

Salabhasana: Locust Pose

Salabhasana, or the "Locust Pose," is often performed in two variations—one following the other. The first is a single-leg Locust Pose, commonly referred to as the "Half Locust Pose" (*ardha-salabhasana*—*ardha* means "half"), followed by a full "Locust Pose" (*salabhasana*). This asana gives a particularly powerful stretch to the entire back of the body, including both the back and the legs. It also helps to tone the buttocks and abdominal organs.

To perform Half Locust Pose, lie flat on your belly on your mat or on a comfortable padded surface, arms at the sides. Your legs and feet should be together and in contact with the ground, your toes pointed behind you. Your chin should be resting on the floor so that the face remains in a neutral position. Make fists with your hands. Gently rock your pelvis and hips from side to side as you slide your fists under your pelvis. Your knuckles are facing toward the ground and the inside surface of your forearms is facing toward the ceiling. If this position is uncomfortable for you, try placing your hands flat on the ground under your pelvis, or hands and arms alongside your body. In whichever variation you choose, extend the fingers so that the hands provide more active support. Let your upper torso remain tight and active.

With an inhalation, slowly contract the right buttock as you extend your right leg and begin to draw it back and up. Initiate the movement from the toes and ball of the feet, as though they are pulling and stretching the leg. Keep your right leg straight and lift it as high as you can while making sure that your left leg remains securely placed on the floor and your hips remain even (see Fig. 13.7a).

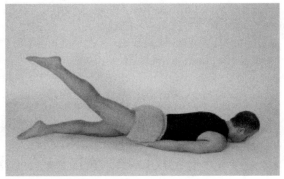

Fig. 13.7a: Half Locust Pose

Hold it in this position for several breaths or longer if it is comfortable. When you are ready to release the leg, exhale and slowly return your right leg to its base starting position.

Repeat Half Locust Pose with your left leg.

If you are a beginner, repeat Half Locust Pose once again on each side of the body. If you are an intermediate practitioner or more advanced, do Half Locust on each side as many times as you wish.

After completing ardha-salabhasana (Half Locust Pose) with each leg, you are ready to execute salabhasana, full, or double-leg, Locust Pose. Begin with the same body placement as for Half Locust: lie flat on your belly; legs and feet together; chin on the floor; fists under your pelvis, or hands under your pelvis or by your sides.

With an inhalation, contract the buttocks muscles and slowly extend both legs

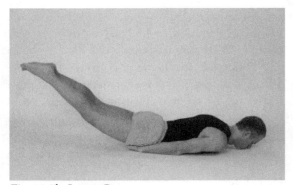

Fig. 13.7b: Locust Pose

and begin to draw them back and up. Your legs and feet are touching. Initiate the movement from the toes and balls of the feet as though they are pulling and stretching the leg. Keep your legs straight and extended and lift them as high as you can. Press down on your hands to allow you to get an extra lift and stretch in the back area, particularly in the lower back (see Fig. 13.7b). Maintain this full Locust Pose for as long as it is comfortable. When you are ready to release from this asana, exhale and slowly return both legs to the floor. Turn your head to one side. Breathe. Rest and relax. You're doing a great job. Take a moment to acknowledge what a great job you're doing

Locust Pose is a powerful backward bending exercise that is often included in a basic yoga practice. You can practice Locust Pose either independently to tone the back and buttocks, or include it in your "Complete Yoga Session" as one of the backward bending exercises, along with, or in place of, the Cobra and Bow Poses.

Knee Hugs: Releases for the Lower Back

As a counterposture to backward bending exercises, it can be nice to massage and release the muscles of the lower back. The following yogic stretch and its variations are ideal for this purpose.

Knees-to-Chest Pose

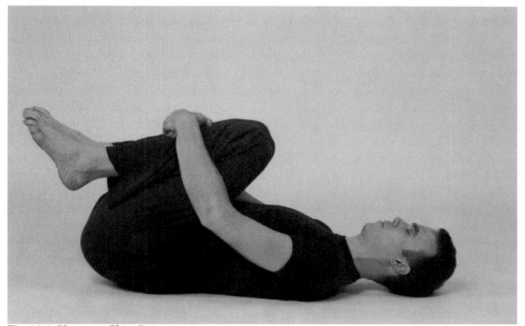

Fig. 13.8: Knees-to-Chest Pose

As a counterpose to the Locust Pose (or any other backward bending exercise), you can do some "knee hugs." Lie comfortably on your back on the floor. Lift your legs off the floor as you bend your knees and hug them into your chest by clasping the area of the upper shins just below the kneecaps with your hands. This Knees-to-Chest Pose is known alternatively as *pavanamuktasana*, *apanasana*, or *vatayanasana* ("Wind-Relieving Pose"). Hold yourself in this position for several complete breaths.

If you would like to deepen the stretch in Knees-to-Chest Pose even further, then lift your head up and bring your forehead as close to your knees as possible. Hug your upper body against your lower body. When you're ready, release your back down to the ground as you continue to hug your knees close to your belly. Gently rock your knees from side to side. Make clockwise circles with your knees, then reverse and make counterclockwise circles. Make "windshield wipers" of your legs as you move them from side to side. Feel the wonderful massage you are giving your lower back and spine. When you are ready, gently begin to rock back and forth on your spine. As you inhale, rock backward onto your spine. As you exhale, rock forward on your spine. Continue massaging your spine with this forward and backward rocking movement for several breaths.

Yoga for Better Urinary and Prostate Health

At some point in their lives, many men experience urinary bladder problems, particularly as they approach middle age. Many men also experience difficulties with the prostate gland—an enlarged prostate gland, prostatitis (inflammation of the prostate gland) and prostate cancer are some of the leading health concerns of today's man. Prostate cancer is now so widespread that it is estimated that up to one-fifth of American men will be diagnosed with prostate cancer at some point in their lives.[4] Prostate cancer is the second leading cause of death from cancer among men, following skin cancer. While prostate cancer can be a deadly disease, modern medicine is making treatment advances. Every man is strongly encouraged to consult with his medical doctor regarding ongoing screening tests for prostate cancer.

Prevention is the best way for a man to avoid having difficulties with the urinary tract and prostate gland. Good diet, exercise, hygiene, and frequent ejaculation are some of the measures that can help keep your urogenital system in top health. In addition, there are specific yoga postures that can help to improve the circulation and range of motion in the pelvic girdle, which has a beneficial health effect on all the organs and glands that are housed there—for men, in particular, the urinary tract, penis, and prostate gland. In addition, a special yogic energy lock that contracts the area of the pelvic floor can help strengthen the muscles that are located there and promote a healthy bladder and prostate. Some yoga asanas that can help you to open your pelvis and groin area, as well as a yogic lock and exercise for the pelvic floor, are included here. Try them out as you give yourself an internal as well as an external workout!

Baddha Konasana: Cobbler Pose

Baddha konasana literally means "Bound Angle Pose" in Sanskrit, but is more commonly referred to as "Cobbler Pose" because it resembles the position in which cobblers in India traditionally sit when they work. This exercise is one of the very best postures in yoga to open a man's hip and groin area. In addition to promoting better bladder and prostate function, it can help the functioning of the kidneys and abdominal organs while stretching the thighs and muscles of the hips and buttocks.

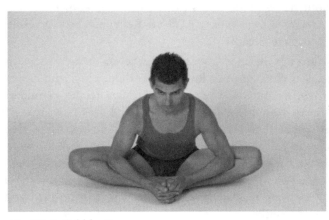

Fig. 13.9: Cobbler Pose

Begin by sitting erect on your sit-bones in a comfortable seated position on the floor, legs straight out and together on the ground in front of you. Sitting on a carpeted or padded surface will provide greater comfort. Place your arms straight down along your sides with your palms pressed into the floor. Press down on your palms to help make your spine even more erect. Slowly flex your legs as you bend them at the knee joint and bring the heels and soles of your feet together in front of you. Bring your heels to within about a foot, or as close as your flexibility permits, to the genital area. Take a moment to be aware of how your legs feel. Do your thighs and knees comfortably touch the ground? If you're like most men, they probably don't. If your knees are raised high off the ground and the posture feels uncomfortable to you, try placing pillows, cushions, blankets, or rolled-up towels under your thighs to support them.

Clasp the top, outside surfaces of the feet with the hands and press firmly inward so that the soles of the feet stay firmly pressed together. Exhale as you bring your upper body forward (see Fig. 13.9). As a variation of Cobbler Pose, you can open the soles of the feet— the outer edges of the feet and heels stay together as the balls of the feet open up like a book, with the soles opening toward the ceiling. In either variation, relax the groin in the direction of the knees, encouraging the hips and thighs to open. Hold Cobbler Pose for up to 30 seconds if you are a beginner. As you progress in this posture, hold the position for one to five minutes.

Supta Baddha Konasana: Reclining Cobbler Pose

Supta baddha konasana, or "Reclining Cobbler Pose" (*supta* means "sleeping" or "reclining") is a variation of the seated Cobbler Pose. This pose can be even more relaxing than the seated Cobbler Pose. In fact, one yoga teacher I know playfully refers to this pose as "Goddess Pose" because of the luxurious sense of relaxation and ease it can give. If you have difficulty sitting on the floor with your back erect, or if you'd like to practice Cobbler Pose in a different way, try Reclining Cobbler Pose.

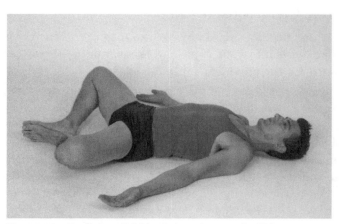

Fig. 13.10a: Reclining Cobbler Pose—Arms at the Sides

To prepare for supta baddha konasana, lie down on a comfortable padded surface on the floor in savasana, or Corpse Pose (see Fig. YPS.3, page 122). Your arms are spread out at equal distance from your sides, palms up.

Your legs are spread out in front of you, your knees are straight, the backs of the legs are in contact with the floor, and your feet are spread out at an equal distance from the midline of the body, slightly wider than hip-width apart. Take a few moments to breathe deeply and rhythmically.

Gradually bend your legs as you slide your feet up so that the soles of your feet meet one another. Bring your feet up, soles still touching, as close to the groin as you comfortably can. Rest the sacrum on the floor to allow the back to maintain its natural alignment. Allow your thighs and knees to open out to the sides as they release toward the floor. Your arms and hands rest on the floor by your sides, palms open and facing the ceiling. You are allowing the force of gravity to work for you in this position—through its effect, gravity is helping your thighs and knees release down toward the floor naturally, opening the hips and thighs even more.

If you would like to go deeper into the pose and give added assistance to gravity, place your hands on your knees or thighs and gently press downward with the hands to increase the stretch (see Fig. 13.10b). Only add this refinement if it is comfortable for you and if it is within your own personal level of comfort and flexibility.

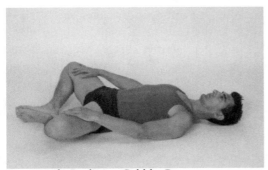

Fig. 13.10b: Reclining Cobbler Pose— Hands on Thighs

Always remember: Yoga is not about competition—with others or yourself. Work within your own edge of comfort. If you are a beginner, hold this pose for up to 30 seconds or so. As you gain experience, hold it for as long as you like.

Reclining Cobbler Pose is a great yoga asana to do when you may just be relaxing at home—even while watching television. Not only will you be deepening your level of relaxation, you'll be doing something very healthy to keep your male organs and reproductive gear in top working order.

Hip Opening Stretch: Ankle Over Raised Knee

This yoga hip opening stretch is one that you can do by itself to help open your pelvis and groin area. You can also incorporate it into your regular workout routine—before or after your workout—as a good stretch for the groin and inner thighs.

Lie on the floor on your back. Bend your knees and place your feet hip-width apart and parallel to one another; soles of the feet on the floor in front of your buttocks. Grasp your left ankle with your two hands and place the ankle in the area of your right thigh that begins just above the knee. Thread your left hand under your left thigh (between your legs) so that it meets your right hand on the back surface of your right thigh. Clasping your right thigh with both hands, gently raise your right foot off the ground, bringing both your legs toward your chest. Hug your right leg in toward your upper body and feel a strong stretch opening up your entire left (and perhaps also right) hip area—thigh, groin, and buttocks.

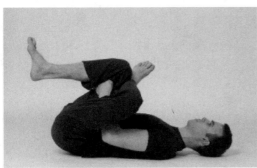

Fig. 13.11: Hip Opening Stretch: Ankle Over Raised Knee

To increase the stretch, try raising your back off the ground as you round your back and bring your head as close to your leg as possible. Hold this stretch for several full rounds of deep, rhythmic breathing. When you are ready to release from the pose, slowly lower your right foot to the ground. Release your hands to your sides as you uncross your legs and place your left foot on the ground, parallel to your right foot. Take a few deep breaths. How do you feel? Does one side of your body feel differently than the other?

Repeat this hip opening stretch on the other side of your body and then slowly stretch your legs, one at a time, out in front of you. Resume Corpse Pose. Rest here for a few minutes while you absorb the benefits of this hip-opening stretch. Take stock of how you feel mentally. Do you feel differently than you did before the stretch—physically, emotionally, and mentally?

Mula Bandha: Pelvic Floor ("Root") Lock

In Sanskrit, the word *bandha* means "lock." In yoga, bandhas are special positions that lock or seal in energy. Yoga practitioners believe that a vital life force energy called *prana* ("air," "breath," or "life force energy" in Sanskrit) runs through the body and sustains us with its life-giving energy. By sealing off certain parts of the body, a man can lock, or trap, the energy inside his body to intensify its vitalizing effects. For this reason, various bandhas are often applied during the exercise of pranayama or meditation to intensify the effect of these yoga practices (see Chapter 16).

Mula bandha is one of these special locks. It is a lock applied to the area of the internal perineum, which is located between the genitals and the anal sphincter. Mula bandha is also sometimes referred to as "Root Lock" because this corresponds to the area where the first, or "root," chakra is believed to lie within the energy system of yoga. The Root Lock is believed to seal in the energy at the base of the spine where the powerful kundalini energy lies coiled. Mula bandha is also sometimes referred to as "Anal Lock" because it involves the contraction of the anal sphincter muscles as well as the surrounding muscles in the pelvic floor.

To begin practicing mula bandha, assume a comfortable cross-legged seated position on the floor or seated in a straight-backed chair. Adjust your alignment so that your sit-bones are firmly rooted on the floor or on the seat of the chair, and your pelvis, shoulders, neck, and head are in a straight line. Bring your attention to the area of the perineum. Contract the muscles that are located in this area, including the sphincter muscles, while you lift up on the area of the perineum. You should feel a gentle pulling in this area.

If you're just beginning to do this exercise, it can be challenging at first. You're becoming sensitive to an area of the body that you may very well generally ignore. As do most men, you've probably become accustomed over time to letting this area function in an involuntary, rather than a voluntary, way.

To assist you in applying this yogic lock, try visualizing a spot about the size of a quarter between your anus and penis, and that a thread suspended from the interior center of your abdominal cavity is gently pulling it up. Allow this imaginary thread to pull this area gently upward as you inhale. Another approach to mastering the anal lock is to practice drawing up on the muscles of the pelvic floor while you are urinating, in order to stop the flow of urine: You are using the muscles that are involved in establishing the Root Lock.

In some approaches to hatha yoga, notably Ashtanga Yoga (see Chapter 6), practitioners are encouraged to apply and maintain the Root Lock without releasing it throughout their entire yoga practice or during portions of it. Accomplished yogis practice applying the yogic lock of mula bandha while sitting in a meditative posture, pressing the heel of the left foot into the groin to contact the area of the perineum, thereby applying pressure to seal the area. They place the right foot on the left leg in what is considered a particularly accomplished pose. They maintain this yogic lock for an extended period of time without releasing it—throughout all of their inhalations and exhalations.

Maintaing Root Lock for extended periods of time in advanced practices is not recommended without qualified supervision and guidance. You can still experiment with using mula bandha while meditating or practicing yogic breathing exercises, however. If you want to take your yoga practice to a new level, try applying mula bandha while you're doing these practices. Just sit in a simple, cross-legged position with your ankles crossed over one another in front of you, apply mula bandha by contracting the muscles of the pelvic floor and hold the contraction throughout your practice while you continue to breathe during your practice. This yogic lock will give you a powerful energy boost in addition to its other valuable male health benefits.

Once you have located the muscles in the pelvic floor and have learned how to contract them in mula bandha, you can incorporate some additional exercises into your health routine. These exercises are related to the Kegel exercises that were developed by a physician to help problems related to urinary incontinence. They can help you to strengthen and tone the muscles of the pelvic floor for improved urinary and prostate health as well as for enhanced sexual control and pleasure.

To practice this set of exercises, begin to exercise the muscles of the pelvic floor by contracting and releasing them. As you inhale, contract the muscles of the pelvic floor, as when applying the Root Lock. Instead of maintaining this contraction for an extended period, however, release these muscles completely on your next exhalation. Then repeat this sequence. Inhale and contract the muscles. Exhale and release them. Continue these pumping, contracting, and releasing movements for about 30 repetitions. Practice this exercise every day, gradually building up to five or more minutes daily. Practicing these exercises is one of the very best practices that you can perform to maintain your prostate, bladder, and reproductive organs in top working order.

Once you feel comfortable practicing these exercises while seated, see if you can do them while standing or performing other activities. Once you master these exercises, you can practice them while you're driving a car, riding the bus to work, or standing in line at the grocery store or bank.

Yoga and Cancer, AIDS, and Other Life-Challenging Concerns

Yoga is by no means a miracle cure—and you should be wary of any healthcare or fitness practitioner who promises a cure to any condition or ailment. However, yoga can offer much comfort to, as well as aid the healing process of, people facing life-challenging illnesses.

One of the most difficult issues facing men with life-threatening illnesses is the fear and lack of control they can feel in their day-to-day lives. Through its ability to calm and still the mind, yoga can help men achieve a place of inner peace, wherein they can see their situation more clearly, without being controlled so deeply by fear. From this place of peace and clarity, a man can be much more able to accept his life condition. A man can see his life more objectively and take positive actions to initiate changes that will help him feel better—both physically and psychologically. Rather than feeling out of control, a man can feel in control. This shift in consciousness is a shift toward healing.

Many health experts believe that positive mental attitudes, such as feeling in control, can help promote healing. Yoga can have other positive health benefits for men, too. Yoga practices can induce the relaxation response and thus help support the functioning of the immune system. This process can help the body to fight and control infection and disease more efficiently. Yoga can also have more subtle effects on a man's health. Once a man embarks on a practice of yoga, he often finds that his life begins to change—subtly and gradually. As he begins to feel good about his body, he wants to take better care of it and spontaneously begins to make lifestyle choices that are healthier and support his well-being, such as stopping health-damaging, addictive behaviors; eating in a more nutritious way; and pursuing healthy exercise.

Adopting just a few simple yogic self-care practices can have a domino effect on initiating other positive changes into a man's life. These lifestyle shifts are factors that can contribute to recovery from illness and disease. Even when yogic practices cannot "cure" an illness, they can help a man to feel better in general, thus reducing the pain and anxiety that accompany many illnesses. And, most important, yoga can help a man to feel whole and at peace with himself—a gift to any man, whether challenged by severe illness or common everyday tribulations.

Yoga for Stress, the Heart, the Mind, and a Host of Other Health Issues

Yoga has become well known as a powerful tool for stress-reduction. Yoga's relation to stress, your heart, and other health issues appears at the end of this chapter because it is meant to underscore and summarize how yoga's ability to reduce stress can support a man as he deals with virtually any health concern he may encounter—from aches and pains to life-threatening challenges. Yoga's power to reduce stress is probably its number-one health benefit.

Yogic practices—the physical postures, yoga meditation, yoga breathing exercises, and the yoga lifestyle in general, including yogic principles of diet—are among the best available today to help combat stress and develop healthy lifestyle habits. While some stress is necessary, and, in fact, desirable, too much stress can be hazardous to a man's health. Indeed, stress seems to be the most pressing and widespread health concern of many men today. Nearly every man complains of life stress—physical stress from physical activity, as well as mental, emotional, and psychological stress at the workplace and in personal relationships with partners, family, and friends.

Stress is intimately connected to illness. In fact, many experts maintain that stress is responsible for as much as 80 percent of all illness today. Stress has been shown to impair the function of the immune system, which makes us even more susceptible to disease. It also inhibits the restorative process of healing and recuperation and accelerates the aging process.

In addition to being directly linked to illness, stress often compounds its adverse effect on health by contributing to the formation of the unhealthy lifestyle habits that many men develop trying to flee it or beat it; for example, overeating, drug and alcohol consumption, smoking, and lack of exercising because of lower energy levels. Medical authorities maintain that up to 90 percent of all illness is caused by stress and lifestyle choices that we make regarding such areas as diet and exercise.

This is the bad news about stress. The good news is that because so much illness is caused by stress and lifestyle choices, a man can make the proactive choice to do something to control and mange the level of stress in his life. He can choose to transform unhealthy habits into habits that support health and well-being.

By reading *Yoga for Men* and beginning a personal practice of yoga, a man can take one of the most positive steps available to turn his life in a healthy direction. Yoga is the perfect practice to help a man reduce stress and improve his health. In fact, many men who practice yoga often report that as an added side benefit of their yoga practice, they develop a deeper awareness of their own bodies and needs so that they naturally and spontaneously begin to make healthier lifestyle choices.

Studies have shown that yogic practices can help to induce what Herbert Benson, M.D., coined the "relaxation response," in his best-selling book of the same title. This relaxation response is an antidote to the fight-or-flight response, which is the excited way in which many men react to stressful situations. The pressures of modern life are sending today's man increasingly into this mode. "Life was stressful before 9-11. It's gotten progressively worse," reports Benson.[5]

In addition to reducing stress, yoga can have other wide-ranging health benefits. Yoga practices can help improve both blood and lymph circulation, thus helping nutrients reach their target cells in the body. Improved circulation helps the body remove toxins more efficiently. Yoga can also improve joint mobility and overall flexibility, which, in turn, makes a man's body less prone to injury.

At the forefront of men's health concerns is cardiovascular disease—the number-one killer of American men today. Yoga has proven to be an effective practice in addressing coronary heart disease, as demonstrated through the clinical work of Dean Ornish, M.D. Dr. Ornish has gained a great deal of public attention, as well as admiration, for his work with patients suffering from cardiovascular disease. His pioneering studies at the Preventive Medicine Research Institute have shown that a comprehensive lifestyle change program consisting of yoga and meditation, diet, exercise, and group support can help to reverse coronary heart disease. Many of the elements that comprise this program are time-honored, integral ingredients of the yoga tradition.

Other scientific studies also indicate that yoga is good for the heart and cardiovascular system. One recent study has shown that the practice of Transcendental Meditation (TM), a practice of yoga meditation techniques, can reverse the buildup of fatty deposits in arterial walls.[6] Early studies by Herbert Benson indicated that the practice of TM could help reduce blood pressure. In fact, Benson's pioneering work in discovering and researching the relaxation response was spurred by his observation of the effects of meditation on practitioners of TM. All of these modern, Western scientific discoveries underscore the tremendous contribution that yoga can make to improving a man's heart and cardiovascular system—something yoga practitioners have known for millennia.

If yoga has so many profound benefits on all the systems of a body, it stands to reason that it can do more than just help build a healthy heart. And, in fact, other scientific studies are beginning to emerge that point to a variety of concrete ways in which yoga can help prevent or alleviate a host of specific ailments, including such widespread and debilitating conditions as asthma, carpal tunnel syndrome, and chronic fatigue syndrome.[7] A 1991 report concluded that clients diagnosed with cerebral palsy who received weekly Phoenix Rising Yoga Therapy sessions became more empowered, self-responsible, and physically able.[8]

Of particular interest to men, and at the cutting-edge of research in male health today, Dr. Ornish believes that yoga may offer special hope for men. In 1997, he and his colleagues at the Preventive Medicine Research Institute began a randomized, controlled study to determine if a comprehensive lifestyle change program including yoga and meditation, dietary modifications, exercise, and group support might slow, stop, or reverse the progression of prostate cancer as measured by PSA (prostate specific antigen), a surrogate marker for prostate cancer progression. Results from the first phase of this Prostate Cancer Lifestyle Trial are encouraging. The study is continuing long-term to assess differences in progression and mortality between the experimental and control groups. The approach to yoga used in both Dr. Ornish's programs for coronary heart disease and in his prostate cancer trial incorporates asanas, deep relaxation, meditation, breathing practices, and visualization to induce relaxation, and, hence, possibly enhance immune system function.

In addition to all the physical health benefits that have been discussed, it is helpful to note that yoga can also be good for a man's mental health and state of mind. Yoga practices can help a man achieve greater balance of body and mind, and to reach a state of calmness where he can become much more in touch with his feelings and emotions. The subject of mental health is far too vast and complex to be summarized here: In the section that follows you'll find suggested resources for further reading if you'd like to explore the subject of yoga psychology in-depth.

So, besides just making you feel good, yoga can be a cornerstone of your ongoing health maintenance routine. Practice yoga regularly and you'll realize for yourself its amazing ability to restore, rejuvenate, strengthen, tone, and improve your overall physical functioning and well-being—body, mind, and spirit.

Suggested Further Resources

If you'd like to find out more about how yoga can help you or a friend or loved one with particular health concerns, the following resources are recommended:

Yoga and Your Back

Books

Mary Pullig Schatz, M.D., et al., *Back Care Basics: A Doctor's Gentle Yoga Program for Back and Neck Pain Relief* (Rodmell Press, 1992). This helpful book, written by a medical doctor and yoga therapist, shows how you can use yoga to relieve back pain. It is complete with illustrated instructions for helpful postures and includes a foreword by yoga master, B.K.S. Iyengar.

Videotapes

Living Yoga—Back Care for Beginners (Healing Arts, 1998). Part of a series of *Living Yoga* tapes produced by Healing Arts, this videotape shows you step-by-step how you can use yoga to improve the health of your back.

Yoga for Your Abs and Butt

Videotapes

Living Yoga's Abs Yoga for Beginners with Rodney Yee (Yoga Journal's Yoga Practice Series), (Healing Arts Publishing, Inc., 1998). Another video in the *Living Yoga* series, this title features Rodney Yee, dubbed the "it boy" of yoga by *USA Today*, presenting 15 minutes of abdominal yoga exercises, along with some breathing, relaxation, and awareness exercises.

Yoga and Your Heart

Dean Ornish, M.D., *Dean Ornish's Program for Reversing Heart Disease: The Only System Scientifically Proven to Reverse Heart Disease without Drugs or Surgery* (Random House, 1990). This is Dr. Ornish's presentation of his revolutionary program for reversing heart disease.

Further information on Dr. Ornish and his work can be found at the following Websites:

www.pmri.org: The Preventive Medicine Research Institute (a nonprofit foundation).

www.ornish.com: Dr. Ornish's Website, with a link to Dr. Ornish's Lifestyle Program at *www.WebMD.com*.

Yoga and a Man's Specific Health Concerns

Yoga approaches have been developed that address the special needs of men who are suffering from specific physical disabilities. For instance, yoga classes for men with AIDS, yoga for those in wheelchairs, and yoga for other special health concerns are offered by many yoga centers and studios. Check to see if your local yoga center or healthcare facility has a class or program available that suits your particular needs.

In addition, B.K.S. Iyengar developed an entire approach to yoga that draws heavily on the use of props and accessories to help people with specific physical challenges perform yoga postures more easily so that they derive therapeutic benefit from them. For more information on Iyengar Yoga, as well as information on how to find an Iyengar Yoga practitioner near you, see Chapter 4.

Integrative Yoga Therapy trains yoga practitioners to deal with specific physical conditions within the traditional healthcare setting. For more information on Integrative Yoga Therapy, see the entry on its approach to yoga in Chapter 10.

The following book deals with how yoga can address specific health concerns:

Larry Payne, et al., *Yoga Rx: A Step by Step Program to Promote Health, Wellness, and Healing for Common Ailments* (Broadway Books, 2002).

Yoga and Your Mental Health

The following books address the relationship of yoga to emotions and the mind:

Swami Ajaya, Ph.D., *Yoga Psychology: A Practical Guide to Meditation* (Himalayan Institute Press, 1976).

Swami Rama and Swami Ajaya, *Creative Use of Emotion* (Himalayan Institute Press, 1976).

Men's Health Resources on the Internet

The Internet is host to an incredibly large and ever-expanding amount of valuable information regarding men's health. In Chapter 17, you'll find information regarding some of the best sites on the Internet for finding out more about men's health, yoga, and other resources helpful to today's man, including some Websites with specific resources regarding prostate health.

Edward S. Goldberg, M.D., on yoga for men's health:

"Yoga has health benefits, especially as it involves circulation and stress reduction. Stress has long been known to be associated with exacerbation of physiologic illnesses such as hypertension, heart disease, diabetes, and many others. Men, in particular, may experience benefit in prevention of cardiac disease, as there is a greater risk of cardiovascular disease in men as compared to women. In addition, increased blood circulation and decrease in stress may impact greatly on prostate health. Chronic prostatitis is associated with aging, stress, and poor circulation, making it a good disease target for prevention with yoga. Musculoskeletal health will also improve with regular physical activity and practice of yoga."

—Edward S. Goldberg, M.D., Physician and Yoga Practitioner

John B. Montana, M.D., on yoga for men:

"Stress is one of the most basic factors that impacts a man's physical, mental, and emotional health. Yoga is one of the best ways to deal with stress. Men facing serious medical conditions can use yoga as a way to gain control and hope in their lives to better cope with their conditions. I've observed that my patients who practice yoga have an inner control, without the use of drugs. I'm also amazed at what good muscle tone these patients have, especially in their core abdominal area. When I palpate their abdominal area, I feel they have the muscle tone of someone who does 40 or 50 sit-ups

(Continued)

a day. In addition to these physical benefits, they have an inner peace that only seems to grow with time."

—John Montana, M.D., Internest specializing in men's health issues

Take a Yoga "Stress-Buster" Break for a Healthy Alternative to Your Coffee Break

While yoga can be practiced in a complete yoga session, you can also use yoga to help restore and renew you nearly anywhere or anytime. Some large commercial airline companies even offer their passengers instructions on "airplane yoga" to help them relax in their seats.

Try taking a Yoga Break as a breather during your day:

■ Sit in a chair and practice some Three-Part Rhythmic Breathing or Alternate Nostril Breathing.

■ Practice some of the stretches from "A Complete Yoga Practice Session for Men"; for instance, Standing Forward Bend.

■ Practice some of the stretches contained in this chapter; for instance, Cat Stretch or Seated Cat Stretch.

■ Take some time to close your eyes and practice meditation—focus on your breathing.

■ Incorporate into your break any of the other yoga practices and techniques that you find especially helpful in this book.

Chapter 14

YOGA AND A MAN'S SEX LIFE

Enhancing Your Sexual Life With Yoga

There is a Persian poem that says, "On the ladder of love, reverence is the first rung leading to the person you love." If a person has no reverence for the beloved one, then he does not have true love.[1]

—Swami Rama

"Yoga and sex?" you might ask. "I thought yogis were spiritual people—into the mind, not the body." If yoga and sex sound like strange bedfellows to you, then you might be surprised to learn that many paths of yoga encourage a healthy respect for sex. In fact, some traditions even encourage the active cultivation of sexual energy and union with a partner to help arouse one's own latent energy—sexual, creative, and spiritual. Perceived in light of yoga, sex can be a way for a man to achieve complete self-realization—of body, mind, and spirit.

When it comes to sex, men in the West are often deeply influenced by the Judeo-Christian tradition that tends to portray sex as something necessary, but accompanied by guilt. In contrast with this tradition is the cultural background of India, where the joy, beauty, and, yes, divinity of sex have been celebrated for thousands of years. Perhaps you've seen photographs of some Hindu temples, such as the spectacular complex of shrines at Khajuaro, which are completely decorated with sculptured reliefs of gods and goddesses in a dizzying array of contorted sexual acts.

Yoga means "union." Nearly every variety in which yoga is practiced has always had the principal goal of uniting man's individual self with the greater universal spirit or principle, known as *Brahman* ("Absolute"). In fact, the two are seen as one and the same in many traditions. Each man is divine. The problem is that his individual ego gets in the way of his realizing this ultimate truth. Yoga practices are designed to help men attain the clear and centered state in which they can see that they are not separate from the universal energy that surrounds them. Once they are able to experience that for themselves, the veil of illusion (*maya* in Sanskrit) that separates them from other beings and objects disappears: They are enlightened.

In order to help men achieve this ultimate union of the individual self with the greater consciousness of the universe, yoga has developed sacred, ritualistic practices to help men achieve union with a sexual partner. In so doing, you are achieving union not just with the limited, individual self of your partner, but also with the divine spirit present within him or her. This union is thus a deep, intimate union that involves not just the physical acts of sexual relationship, but also a true merging of souls.

Nearly all yoga practices can help you enjoy a better sex life. The physical postures of yoga will make you stronger and fitter, and so better able to enjoy the physical pleasures of lovemaking. Meditation and breathing practices will help you be more centered, and consequently, more present during the act of lovemaking: Making love can then become more enjoyable both for you and your partner. Yoga will also help you to feel more relaxed, thus helping to eliminate stress related to performance anxiety and its potential attendant disorders. You may find as a result of your yoga practice that some common sexual problems—such as premature ejaculation, difficulty with erections or with orgasm, and even issues related to impotence—spontaneously disappear as yoga helps you become more centered, relaxed, and present.

In regard to particular yogic sexual practices, there is a path of yoga that has evolved and developed specific sexual practices as part of its path to enlightenment. This is the path of *tantra*—a term you may have heard. There is much information currently available about tantra, but there is also a great deal of confusion, so it is worthwhile to take a look at this tradition of yoga practices in greater depth.

Tantra: A Wide Web of Practices

Tantra is a Sanskrit word that literally means "loom" and is associated with weaving. Tantric yoga is an approach to yoga that developed to help men achieve self-realization by weaving their own individual selves with the greater cosmic Self. Sexual tantric practices can help a man to achieve self-realization by sexually weaving himself in a sacred union with a sexual partner.

The origins of tantra are obscure, although some scholars believe its roots are very ancient and formed part of both Hindu and Buddhist traditions. Because it is comprised of many and varied practices, it is difficult to define Tantrism in simple terms. According to some, Tantrism flourished most fully from 500 to 700 C.E., and represented an alternative to traditional yoga practices, which had, until then, been reserved for the priestly class in India. Tantric yoga allowed ordinary laypersons to practice yoga.[2]

For many men, tantric yoga is synonymous with sexual yoga. However, sexual practices make up a relatively small part of tantra—about only 10 percent, according to some authorities. The majority of tantric yoga is devoted to mantra recitation, or the recital of certain sacred sounds, as a way of weaving the individual self with divinity.[3]

Tantrism pays tribute to the sacred divine feminine principle of cosmic energy known as *shakti*. A basic precept behind the sexual practices of tantric yoga is that each man and woman is divine. By recognizing and worshiping the divine principle in your sexual partner, you can come closer to achieving unity with the divine. This union is characterized by a deep spiritual connection, not just the physical release of orgasm. In fact, in some esoteric sexual practices, men are encouraged to explore and enjoy their sexual energy without having an orgasm with ejaculation. In many Eastern traditions, it is a commonly held belief that men are born with a fixed, predetermined store of vital energy. Each ejaculation results in the discharge of some of this energy, leading to physical decline.

Tantric yoga can help a man send energy from the area of his sexual organs to higher energy centers, such as those of the heart and mind. The practices of tantric yoga are intimately related to kundalini yoga. Kundalini yoga attempts to awaken the divine feminine energy that resides in each individual—man and woman—in the form of kundalini-shakti, where it lies stored at the base of the spine. Awakening this latent energy can help a man achieve self-realization (see Chapter 7). The divine feminine principle is believed to exist not only in human beings, but it also pervades the entire universe, and is the source of all of creation. In some approaches to tantric practices, a man can cultivate the arousal of this creative energy by igniting and maintaining his sexual energy at heightened levels for prolonged periods of time without ejaculating.

Tantric yoga in the West has become interwoven with a host of other practices. If you are thinking of attending a class, workshop, or retreat in practices advertised as tantric yoga, the old adage applies: "Buyer Beware." Some teachers of tantric yoga are steeped in the Indian tradition of tantra, with many years of training and experience; however, many teachers of tantric yoga are really putting together a number of ingredients from a variety of practices—bodywork, psychotherapy, and the human potential movement—and applying the now generic and trendy term of tantric yoga to their work.[4] So if you'd like to explore tantric yoga classes or programs, find out beforehand what the one you are interested in actually entails. Some tantric yoga classes may include explicit training in various tantric erotic practices. Others may focus on the teachings and philosophy of tantra. Others may be geared more toward opening your heart so that you are more fully able to give and receive love.

A Tantric Ritual

Many men today are extremely tense. In their relationships with their partners, their focus is often on immediate gratification of their sexual needs. Their partners may end up performing out of a sense of obligation, and the end result can be frustration for both parties. By becoming more relaxed and open, a man can help nurture a sense of deep trust in his relationship with his partner. This sense of trust can not only help to improve the quality of a man's sexual life, but it can also spill over into all of his relationships.

Tantric yoga with a sexual partner involves worshiping the divinity of your partner. It is about being open and giving of yourself to please your partner in every way that you can—tactilely, sensorially, emotionally, and spiritually. It is about complete giving and abandonment without thinking about receiving. For, according to tantra, in giving of your entire self you will receive far more than you ever imagined possible.

So try performing a tantric ritual of your own. Set aside an evening or a special time where you will do nothing but be attentive and responsive to your partner's needs—whether your partner is female or male. Set a special atmosphere—light candles, arrange flowers in a vase, play soft music, burn some incense, or diffuse fragrant essential oils. Prepare or have available some special delicacies for your partner. Draw a bath for your lover and bathe him or her gently. Sit across from your partner and stare into his or her eyes, merging your souls. Let the energy of your heart center extend across the space between you to kiss your partner's heart center. Spend hours making love, placing your entire emphasis on your partner. Become aware of how you feel when you give freely without worrying about receiving. You might want to prearrange another time when your partner can reciprocate so that you are the recipient. See how you feel in this situation.

You may be surprised to learn how enjoyable and gratifying it can be to be totally absorbed in giving. Because your attention is single-pointedly focused on your partner, you are, in fact, performing a kind of meditation. The meditative, totally present state in which you find yourself can be one that is calming and blissful. In addition, you can relax about your own performance. If you're not worried about whether you're getting what you want out of the sexual arrangement, you'll most likely not feel disappointed or resentful if your needs are not met. Now, just for this period of time, you have no needs or expectations. And if you don't focus on orgasm as your be-all and end-all, you may find that any performance anxieties spontaneously disappear. Indeed, you may even discover, as a result of performing this tantric ritual, that you harbored some unconscious performance anxieties that only surfaced when you became totally present and mindful.

In this tantric ritual, you don't have to perform. You don't have to ejaculate. All you have to be is totally, undividedly present for your partner. And in this undivided state of union with your beloved, you have an opportunity to experience the bliss that flows from the true realization of your self.

Yoga to Enhance Your Sexual Performance

Maybe a tantric yoga ritual isn't for you. Maybe you're not worried about shortening your life through multiple orgasms and ejaculations. Maybe you're just wondering if yoga can help you get more out of your sex life.

The answer is *yes*: Yoga can help you have a better sex life, too. The practice of yoga, in general, will help to make your body stronger and more flexible, your heart healthier, and your breathing deeper and fuller—all of which can help make your lovemaking more ardent and more passionate. In addition, yoga can help to make your mind more relaxed and open to receiving the pleasures of sex. It can also help to reduce anxieties you may have about your performance in the bedroom.

Certain yoga asanas and practices are especially helpful for promoting the optimal functioning of a man's reproductive organs. Not surprisingly, many of these emphasize opening, stretching, and strengthening the areas of the buttocks, hips, and pelvis.

One of the very best yoga practices for strengthening and toning the urogenital area is applying the yogic lock of mula bandha, described in Chapter 13. Practicing the allied Kegel exercises (contracting and releasing the muscles of the pelvic floor) is one of the best exercises you can do to increase sexual stamina and performance. In many books on tantric yoga, you may see Kegel exercises referred to as PC exercises—"PC" stands for "pubococcygeus" and refers to a group of muscles that surround the penis and anus.[5] In addition to massaging the prostate gland, Kegel, or PC, exercises can help strengthen the muscles in the genital area, bring increased circulation and blood to your sexual organs, help you build more stamina and control when making love, and, some men claim, even make you shoot farther when you do ejaculate.[6] These exercises can also help you become more aware of your sex organ and be more sensitive to the pleasurable sensations you experience when you make love. Additional yoga postures presented in Chapter 13 that can help open your pelvic area and improve your sexual performance and enjoyment include both Seated and Reclining Cobbler Pose (see Fig. 13.9 and 13.10a and b).

Additional yoga postures you might want to try to spice up your sex life are Pigeon Pose and Eagle Pose. Pigeon Pose gives a deep stretch to the hips, pelvis, and groin for increased ease and openness in this area. Eagle Pose is touted by some practitioners of yoga as one of the best yogic positions for increasing sexual stamina. Bikram Choudhury, yogi to the superstars, is reported to have boasted that Eagle Pose is great for sex: "You can make love for hours and have seven orgasms when you are 90."[7] Choudhury is known for his tendency to overstate: Try Eagle Pose for yourself and see what it does for your sex life whether you're 90 or not. Directions for performing both Pigeon Pose and Eagle Pose follow.

Kapotasana: Pigeon Pose

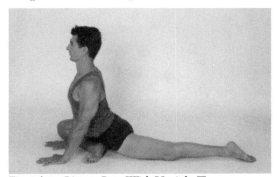

Fig. 14.1a: Pigeon Pose With Upright Torso

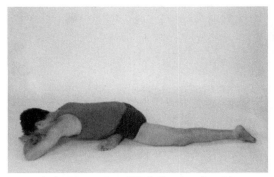

Fig. 14.1b: Pigeon Pose With Forehead on Floor

Kapotasana, or "Pigeon Pose," is one of the best yoga asanas for opening the hip and buttocks area. Many men are tight in this area, resulting in restricted mobility in the pelvic girdle.

One of the easiest ways to enter into Pigeon Pose is from Downward-Facing Dog (see Fig. YPS.1j, page 118). To prepare for Pigeon Pose, kneel on the floor on all fours with your arms under your shoulders and your knees under your hips. Press the palms and fingers of your hands into the floor and curl your toes under your feet. Straighten your legs and lift up your tailbone to assume Downward-Facing Dog.

Your body now forms an inverted V relative to the floor. Straighten your right leg and extend it up and back as far behind you as you comfortably can. Bend the right knee as you bring it close to your forehead as you round your neck and release your head toward the floor. Release your right leg to the floor by bending your right knee and placing the front surface of your left leg straight on the floor. Your right knee is now positioned forward between your hands. Slide the right foot toward the left side of your body. The heel of the right foot is now beneath your belly or pelvis. Lift your chest and heart center to maintain your torso upright. Support your upper body with your fingertips or palms pressing into the floor (see Fig. 14.1a).

If you would like to vary the stretch in Pigeon Pose, lower your upper body toward the floor. Place your forehead on the floor. You can either stretch your arms out in front of you or rest your forehead on the backs of your hands (see Fig. 14.1b).

When you are ready to release from Pigeon Pose, lengthen and raise your upper body to an upright position. Shift your body over to the right side as you slide your legs out from under you so that they are now in front of you. Wiggle the legs from side to side, and repeat Pigeon Pose on the other side of the body.

Garudasana: Eagle Pose

Garudasana, or "Eagle Pose," is a traditional yoga pose that you can use to help increase your sexual energy. To prepare for Eagle Pose, assume an erect standing position as in Mountain Pose (see Fig. YPS.1a, page 115). Your feet are parallel to one another and about hip-width apart. Shift your weight to your left leg for support as you lift up your right leg. Lift and wrap the right thigh over the left thigh and hook the right foot or toes behind the left calf. If necessary, use your hands to help hook your right leg into position. If this is too challenging, then simply lift and wrap your right thigh over the left thigh and let your right foot and toes hang out to the side of your left leg. As you perform Eagle Pose, you will be forming a slight crouching position as your abdomen moves back and your hips move forward. Now cross the elbows in front of you with the elbow of your left arm crossing over the inside crease of the elbow of your right arm. Double-cross your arms so that you can press your palms together and lift your elbows to shoulder height so that the upper arms are parallel to the floor and your

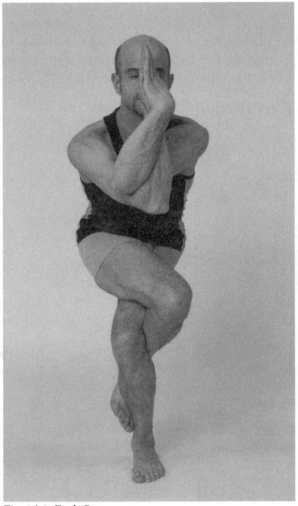

Fig. 14.2: Eagle Pose

forearms are perpendicular to the floor. If you can, fold forward so that your arms are in front of your knees and your forearms extend beyond your legs to form a 90-degree angle to the floor (see Fig. 14.2). Hold this position for several breaths if you are a beginner and for longer if you are more experienced. To come out of the position, slowly unwrap your arms, then your legs, and return to Mountain Pose, standing erect with your feet parallel to one another and inside edges touching.

Now prepare to repeat Eagle Pose on the other side of your body.

Once you have performed Eagle Pose on both sides of the body, take a moment to be mindful of how you feel. Do you feel any differently, especially in the groin, pelvis, and hip areas?

Eagle Pose is one of the most challenging postures in *Yoga for Men*. The model illustrating this pose is especially accomplished. Do whatever you can and whatever feels comfortable. If you find Eagle Pose difficult to maintain on the first few tries, don't be discouraged. With regular practice, you will get better. You may feel a bit like a human pretzel doing this particular yoga posture, but the twisting and strengthening of the central core area of your body can result in beneficial results not only for your sex life, but also for your entire being.

The Fast Track to Enlightenment: "Cut" to the Heart

"Free yourself from all fears" is the first message of the Himalayan sages.[8]

—Babaji instructing Swami Rama

Yoga is not only a physical practice, but also a rich body of knowledge that flows from a tradition of perennial spiritual wisdom. If you were to distill the essence of the spiritual wisdom that informs this tradition, you would come to a few simple principles that explain the dynamics of a man's existence and his reason for being: Man is trapped by fear. He may have many fears but, ultimately, all fears are a reflection of a man's fear of his mortality. Because of fear, men become trapped and limited in their way of thinking and being. The path of yoga is a path of awareness that leads to seeing our fears as groundless because we are not our fears. We are more than our fears: We are limitless beings. When a man is able to comprehend this basic truth, his soul becomes light and his heart opens. The opening of the heart is one of the best ways to let go of fear. Once the heart is open, a man's mission in life becomes clear: to serve humanity in whatever form that may take. It doesn't mean becoming a renunciant—it can simply mean serving others in the best way you are able, whether you are a carpenter, bank teller, or CEO.

For this reason, yoga has always placed special emphasis on the opening of the heart. Indeed, many of the physical postures of yoga help to open the torso—and, in particular, the chest and heart area. Many of the tantric yoga workshops offered in the West focus on the area of the genitals, aiming to stimulate the flow of energy there. But true tantric yoga practice in the spiritual tradition that was first laid down centuries ago focuses on the area of the heart, aiming to open and soften the heart so that we are free to give and to receive loving energy in perfect union not only with our sexual partner, but with all that the universe has in store for us.

To take the fast track to yoga enlightenment, concentrate on opening your heart. Don't work at it; simply allow it to happen as you surrender your soul. If you'd like to support the opening of your heart with some asanas drawn from hatha yoga practice, try doing some postures that open the chest fully. Poses in "A Complete Yoga Practice Session for Men" that are good heart openers include the back bending Cobra Pose (Fig. YPS.8) and Bow Pose (Fig. YPS.9). Triangle Pose (Fig. YPS.4a and b) also helps to open the heart.

Many men have closed chests, with shoulders that are rounded forward. Prominent reasons for this are poor posture and sitting hunched in front of computers and desks. Even weightlifters that don't combine complete stretching routines with their bodybuilding are working to close off their chest areas. As men develop those much-admired pectoral muscles, they are also tightening the musculature of the chest area and causing the shoulders to round forward. This tightening of the chest area creates armor around a man's heart. The tendency to close off the chest area physically only seems to grow as we get older. So to help open your chest area—and your heart—try the following yoga exercise.

Standing Forward Bend With Arms Raised Overhead and Behind

Doing the following variation on the Standing Forward Bend will help to open your heart, as well as help stretch out your chest area after a day of sitting stooped over a desk at the office.

Assume an erect standing position, such as Mountain Pose (Fig. YPS.1a, page 115). Separate your feetso that they are parallel and hip-width apart. Keeping your arms straight, move them back behind you. Bring your palms together and interlace your fingers behind your back. Inhale as you arch your chest and the front of your pelvic basin forward, letting your neck roll gently backward so that your nose tilts toward the ceiling. (If you experience any neck problems, be careful not to arch your neck back too far.) Keep your arms as straight as possible, and, if you can, your palms pressed against one another throughout the remainder of the exercise. If this is too difficult for you, then simply interlock your fingers together without palms touching. Exhale as you bend forward from the hips allowing your upper

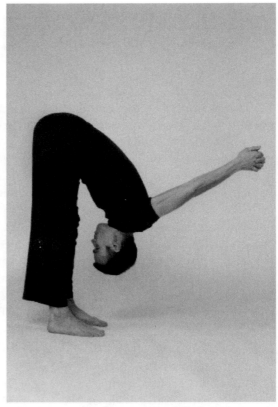

Fig. 14.3: Standing Forward Bend With Arms Raised Overhead and Behind

body and head to lower toward the floor. As you lower your upper body, press your arms and hands out in back from you and away from your body, keeping your arms as straight as possible. Rotating your arms from the shoulders, press your hands as far in back of you as you can, then up toward the ceiling, and, if possible, out over your back so that they are pointing in front and away from your body (see Fig. 14.3). Breathe several full, deep rhythmic breaths in this position. Feel your heart center opening and expanding as your chest, shoulders, and even armpits expand and widen. To come out of this pose, inhale as you gently raise your upper body back to a full standing position while releasing your arms down along the sides of your body. Come back to Mountain Pose. Take several deep breaths in Mountain Pose as you take the time to be aware of how you feel. In particular, bring your awareness to your heart and chest area. In Sanskrit, this posture is referred to as *uttanasana*, or "intense stretch." How do you feel after this intense heart-opening stretch? Do you feel more open and expanded? Does your breathing feel different? Do you feel different? Do you perhaps feel more open to life's possibilities?

This is a simple yet powerful yoga pose that you can incorporate into your daily work life. It's a great exercise to do at work. Take a few minutes every now and then during the day to open your heart and stretch out your chest with this powerful yogic forward bend.

Meditation: Letting Go of Fear/Opening the Heart

Sexual union is about much more than the physical orgasm: It is about being completely open to giving and receiving. Many men have closed off their hearts without even realizing it because of the accumulated unconscious fears that they are holding onto.

The following meditation will help you to see and release your fears. It will help you to open up to give and receive love fully. And then you will be able to participate joyously, completely, and with perfect presence in union not only with your own soul but also with your sexual partner and other people with whom you are intimate in your life.

Try doing this meditation in a quiet place where you will not be disturbed. Because you will be focusing on opening the heart chakra, you may want to precede this meditation with some physical hatha yoga postures to open the heart, such as the forward bending exercise given on page 116, or Bow Pose (see Fig. YPS.9, page 129).

When you are ready to begin the meditation, find a comfortable padded surface on the floor where you can lie down on your back and stretch out comfortably. Dim the lights. Make sure that you will not be interrupted for at least 15 to 20 minutes. Unplug your phone or turn the volume down on your answering machine. Let your family members or roommates know that you don't want to be disturbed while you're practicing this meditation. Have a blanket nearby in case your body becomes cool during the relaxation portion of this meditation. Also, have some pillows, cushions, or rolled-up towels to place under the back of your head and/or knees to make you more comfortable.

Assume a comfortable position lying on the floor on your back in Corpse Pose (see Fig. YPS.3, page 122). The backs of your legs are in contact with the floor, your legs spread out about hip-width or a little further apart, your toes pointing away from your body. Your buttocks, back, and the back of your head are all in comfortable contact with the floor. Your arms are spread several inches out from your body, the backs of your arms in contact with the floor, palms opened toward the ceiling.

Take a few deep, complete yogic breaths, filling up your abdomen, chest, and shoulders with each inhalation, and releasing your breath fully with each exhalation. Now, on an inhalation through your nose, tense your body: Make fists of your hands, tense your buttocks and legs, your pectorals, and even your face. Make your face into a prune. Hold your breath, and then exhale through the mouth. Repeat this contraction/relaxation exercise several times. By contracting and tensing your body and then releasing it, you are making yourself even more open and receptive. Feel this abandon in every cell of your body. Surrender yourself to the floor.

Now bring your awareness to your heart center, a point in the middle of your chest at the level of your heart. Feel a small, bright, white light emanating from your heart center. If you have trouble visualizing a white light, then just feel as though your chest is being filled with light. Feel this light growing larger and expanding out to fill up your entire chest cavity.

Now take the time to witness what is present in your heart. Imagine that you are entering a closet that is full of all kinds of things that you've been putting in there during your entire life. Feel what fears and anxieties fill your heart area. Be aware of them. Don't judge them or criticize them. Just be aware of them. Realize that you don't need to hold on to these fears any longer, and let go of them. You don't need them. Say to them, "I acknowledge and bless you, and release you." Be aware of how your heart center feels. Does it feel fuller, more open, and lighter? Now be aware of what good things are being held in your heart closet. Are there positive qualities you've been developing all your life that are contained in your heart? Compassion? Generosity? Respect for other people? Acknowledge the life-affirming qualities of your heart center and bless them. Feel the love that fills your heart center. Let this love radiate out to your entire being so that you become a being of light, radiating love from your heart center, like rays from the sun. Let this love bathe and bless you. This is your true nature. This is your true self. This is your inner being of light.

Take the time to extend this love outward. If you have a partner or mate, allow this energy of love to stream out from your heart to her or him. If you're not in a romantic relationship with anyone at this time, then let this love radiate out to someone whom you feel could use some love right now, perhaps even to the planet itself. Radiate and send this healing love to the object of your intention.

When you've finished radiating out this love, bring your awareness back to your heart center. Take a moment to gently shut the door of your heart closet to protect you, but leave it ever so slightly ajar so that you can continue to radiate your love.

Rest in blissful repose for as long you like. Bask in your true nature.

When you're ready to return to the here and now, gently wiggle your fingers and toes. Stretch your arms and legs, like a child who is awakening. Be aware of how you feel. Gently roll onto your right side, legs bent and knees stacked on one another in fetal position. Rest here for several breaths. When you are ready, gently roll over onto all fours and slowly round up to standing, keeping your knees bent as you round up to protect your lower back.

Meditating on the heart is a very powerful way for a man to awaken to his full being. Practice this meditation as often as you like. See how it changes your life.

Suggested Further Resources

If you'd like to find out more about tantric yoga and how you can use yoga to enhance your sexual life, the following books are recommended:

Books

Margot Anand, *Sexual Ecstasy: The Art of Orgasm* (J.P. Tarcher, 2000). If you're interested in learning how to give your partner magnificent orgasms, then this fully illustrated guide by one of the most well-known teachers of sexual yoga may be for you.

Pala Copeland and Al Link, *Soul Sex: Tantra for Two* (Career Press, 2003). Written by a couple that has been practicing and teaching tantric yoga for many years, this book shows both beginners and skilled tantric practitioners how to use the techniques of tantra to create lifelong, loving relationships.

Kerry Riley with Diane Riley, *Tantric Secrets for Men: What Every Woman Will Want Her Man to Know about Enhancing Sexual Ecstasy* (Destiny Books, 2002). This book aims to present everything a man needs to know to be a good lover, including practical and easy-to-follow tantric rituals and sacred sexuality exercises for a modern man's lifestyle.

Nik Douglas and Penny Slinger, *Sexual Secrets: The Alchemy of Ecstasy, 20th Anniversary Edition* (Inner Traditions, 2000). Drawing on the wisdom tradition of ancient texts, this now classic and profusely illustrated reference explains how you can use sexuality to achieve the transcendental experience of unity and ecstasy.

The Kama Sutra, or "Rules of Love," is one of the most ancient and well-known guides to lovemaking. Many editions of this book, most based on the 1883 translation into English by Sir Richard Burton, are available. Check your library or a bookstore.

Richard Freeman on yoga for men:

"Yoga involves rhythmical movement and awareness along the central axis of the body. This includes and sublimates sexual function and movement."

—Richard Freeman, a student of yoga since 1968, is Director of the Yoga Workshop in Boulder, Colorado

Chapter 15

PARTNERED YOGA

Yoga Exercises, Stretches, and Poses You Can Do With a Friend, Lover/Spouse, Family Member, Coworker, or Workout Partner

In Partner Yoga, the notion of yoga as union becomes a lived experience as we realize that all souls are one.

—Noll Daniel, Yoga Teacher of Soul-to-Soul Yoga

Yoga is not necessarily just for the individual man. It can also be for two men, or a man and a woman, or even three or more people. Performing partnered yoga can be a truly fun and exciting way to take your practice to a new level. Partnered yoga can provide you with the opportunity of sharing your yoga practice in direct contact with another person. In addition, practicing yoga with the support of another person who can actively coach you into yoga poses can help you stretch further both physically and psychologically, so you can take your yoga practice to a whole new level.

You can practice yoga with any partner of your choosing. If you practice yoga with a sexually intimate partner, it can help you to take your level of closeness to an even deeper and richer level as you help one another explore your inner depths as well as your outer boundaries. You can also practice partnered yoga with a friend or family member for the sheer joy and adventure of it. Or you can choose to try some partnered yoga exercises with your workout buddy to help you both take your workouts to new highs. When sharing yoga with others, the possibilities are virtually endless.

Nearly any yoga posture can be done with a partner. In one common approach to partnered yoga, frequently referred to as Partner Assisted Yoga, one partner serves as a supportive coach to another partner. The second (assisting) partner does not perform the yoga posture him- or herself, but rather helps the first (assisted) partner go deeper into the pose. If the second partner understands the direction in which the first partner is moving in a particular yoga posture, the second partner can apply firm, yet gentle, pressure to help the first partner stretch even deeper into the pose. For instance, in a Seated Forward Bend (see Fig. YPS.6, page 125), the second partner could apply pressure to the first partner's back as the first partner folds the torso forward, thus allowing the first partner to stretch even longer, and closer to the legs and feet.

In another popular approach to partnered yoga, two or more yoga practitioners perform yoga postures simultaneously; thus, supporting one another and receiving the benefits of the partnering at the same time. This approach to yoga practice is often referred to simply as Partner Yoga.

You can experiment with your favorite poses to see how Partner Assisted and Partner Yoga can enhance your yoga practice. To get you started, the following are a few suggestions for some partnered yoga exercises that address virtually all the major areas of the body. They are a good point of embarkation on your journey into exploring yoga with a partner. The illustrations show how a man can do yoga with a male or a female partner.

Partner Assisted Yoga: Getting Started

To begin your journey in partnered yoga, try practicing some of the yoga postures presented in "A Complete Yoga Practice Session for Men" while assisting or being assisted by a partner. This will help to give you a full-body yoga workout and also help you to see how the principles of Partner Assisted Yoga are put into action. The following are representative examples of how you can incorporate the principles of Partner Assisted Yoga into the practice of some basic yoga asanas. Once you see how you can assist, or be assisted by, a partner, you can continue on your own to invent and experiment with your own variations of assisted partnering. You can also check out the Website given at the end of this chapter for further information on suggestions for partnering in specific asanas.

So, pick a partner and start to have some fun!

Adho Mukha Svanasana: Downward-Facing Dog Pose

Adho mukha svanasana, or "Downward-Facing Dog Pose," is one of the most beneficial and commonly practiced yoga asanas. It is deeply calming and restorative. It stretches and strengthens virtually every part of the body: hands, arms, shoulders, back, thighs, lower legs, and even the feet and toes. Because you are in an inverted position while performing Downward-Facing Dog, it also helps to improve circulation and relieve pressure on the internal organs. The stretch it gives to the back can help to counter roundness in the back. Because the upper and lower extremities of your body are bearing weight, this pose can help to build stronger bones. Downward-Facing Dog forms an important part of the Sun Salutation series presented in "A Complete Yoga Practice Session for Men (see Fig.YPS.1j, page 118). Assisting a partner in this physically challenging posture can help the partner go even further into this powerful stretch. Fig. 15.1a and 15.1b show how you can assist a partner from behind while he or she is performing Downward-Facing Dog Pose.

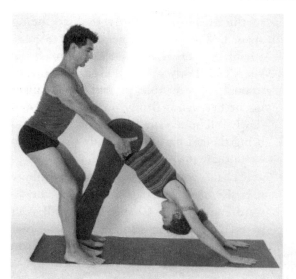

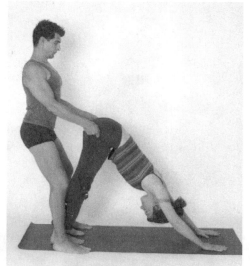

Fig. 15.1a: Downward-Facing Dog With Partner
Lifting Thighs and Pelvis

Fig. 15.1b: Downward-Facing Dog With
Partner Assistance Using a Yoga Strap

Have your partner kneel on all fours on the floor, hands parallel and shoulder-width apart, palms firmly planted on the ground, fingers spread wide for support, and index fingers parallel to one another. Your partner's feet are parallel and hip-width apart. On an exhalation, your partner lifts the knees up off the floor as he or she raises and tilts the pelvis forward. Your partner stretches out the legs so that they are straight, bending the knees as much as is needed if the position is uncomfortable in any way. Your partner takes several rounds of deep, full breaths. Encourage your partner to press his or her heels as close to the ground as possible. Encourage your partner to lift the tailbone even higher as he or she spreads the shoulders wide, crown of the head facing toward the floor. Your partner presses down into the floor firmly with the palms of the hands while lifting the pelvis up, giving a complete stretch to the entire body, from fingers to toes.

With Partner Assisted Yoga, you can help your partner to develop even greater power in Downward-Facing Dog. Stand behind your partner and firmly wrap your hands in the folds between your partner's hips and pelvis. Apply a firm traction to your partner's pelvis, helping to lift it up and back (see Fig. 15.1a). For additional traction, you can take a yoga belt or strap and wrap it around the front of your partner's thighs and lift backward and up (see Fig. 15.1b). Pull firmly on the strap or belt, but only within the level of stretch that is comfortable to your partner. (If the belt feels as though it is pressing too tightly or is otherwise uncomfortable to your partner, then don't do this variation.) As you help your partner to lift his or her lower abdomen and legs, have your partner press his or her hands firmly into the ground to give a complete stretch to both the upper and lower body.

You can also assist a partner to stretch further in Downward-Facing Dog by standing in front of your partner with your feet outside of his or her hands. Place your hands on your partner's sacrum and press in the direction of the sit-bones to bring more length to the area. This variation of Partner Assisted Yoga is illustrated in Fig. 15.1c.

In either variation, as you assist your partner in deepening Downward-Facing Dog, encourage your partner to take full, rhythmic breaths to send fresh, rich oxygenated blood

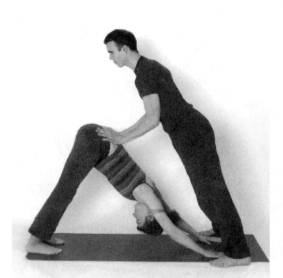

Fig. 15.1c: Downward-Facing Dog With Partner Placing Hands on the Sacrum

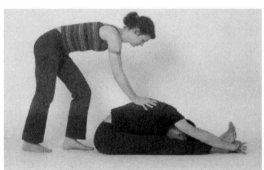

Fig. 15.2: Partner Assisted Seated Forward Bend

to the areas of the body that are being opened. When your partner is ready to come out of the pose, have him or her bend the knees and slowly walk the hands and fingers toward the feet. Your partner should place his or her hands firmly on the thighs and slowly roll up to standing, the neck and head being the last parts of the body to return to an upright position.

Thank your partner for the opportunity to assist him or her in performing Downward-Facing Dog. Change roles with your partner, as he or she assumes the role of providing assisted support as you perform Downward-Facing Dog Pose.

Paschimottanasana: Seated Forward Bend

Paschimottanasana, or "Seated Forward Bend" (Fig. YPS.6, page 125), is one of the best overall stretches for the back and the hamstrings—the long, often tense, muscles that run along the entire length of the back of the upper leg. In this posture, you will assume the position for Seated Forward Bend and execute the posture while your partner assists you in deepening your stretch.

Sit on the floor with your trunk, neck, and head erect with your legs straight out in front of you, touching. Place the palms of your hands firmly pressing into the ground at your sides to ensure that you are sitting as straight as possible. In turn, gently lift each of your buttocks off the floor as you use your hands to spread the tissue in the gluteal area away from the midline of the body: This will help you to sit as directly as possible on your sit-bones. Raise you arms overhead. As you exhale, slowly lower your arms toward your feet. Take hold of your feet or legs with your hands at whatever point you are able to reach most comfortably. Try not to round your back, but rather fold at your hip creases, like a hinge. Take several deep, full breaths.

Your partner can help you get an even stronger stretch in this position. Your partner stands or kneels behind you, facing your back. Your partner can begin by gently massaging your back, moving his or her hands up from your lower back toward your shoulders. When your partner locates the area of your back that feels tightest, your partner places his or her hands on that area of your back, hands alongside the spine (see Fig. 15.2). Your partner should avoid placing any direct pressure on the spine itself. Pressing firmly into your back within your level of comfort, your partner helps you to extend your spine and torso even longer. Your upper body and face will most likely come closer to your legs—perhaps even to the point where they rest directly on your legs. Try to keep your legs straight, but not locked, at the knees. Hold onto your feet if you can; if not, place your hands wherever they most comfortably reach. If necessary, bend your knees as much as you need to. Breathe several full deep breaths in this position.

Paschimottanasana literally means "intense stretch of the west." In Eastern thought, the back is considered the western part of the body. It relates to our past, to all the baggage we have acquired during our lives and are still carrying around with us. No wonder we develop such back pain! Use this opportunity of support and trust offered by your partner to let go of some of this baggage. Mentally say that you don't need to carry around the baggage of the past. Let go. Surrender into the pose as your back opens and breathes, like a newborn. Stay in this position for as long as you like. Take advantage of the luxury of having a partner assist you in going even deeper into your own release than you could do if you were practicing Seated Forward Bend on your own. Thank your partner for this support.

When you are ready to come out of the pose, on an inhalation, round your back up as you return to a full upright sitting position. Take a few deep breaths. Feel the opening that has taken place.

Change roles with your partner: Now he or she performs Seated Forward Bend and you provide assisted support.

Dhanurasana: Bow Pose

Dhanurasana, or Bow Pose (Fig. YPS.9, page 129), is a powerful backward bend. You can help your partner open the back and shoulder area even wider and further than your partner could do on his or her own.

Have your partner lie down on his or her belly on a firm, padded surface. Your partner bends the legs, raising the lower legs off the ground, and lifting the feet toward the buttocks. Your partner grasps the ankles with his or her hands. As your partner inhales, he or she raises the knees and thighs off the ground by lifting up and pulling back on the ankles. As your partner's thighs come off the ground, he or she also lifts the head and front upper torso off the ground, back arching into a backbend. Encourage your partner to breathe deeply and fully during this pose.

You can help your partner deepen the stretch to the muscles of the back and shoulders. Stand behind your partner, facing him or her. Your feet and legs are

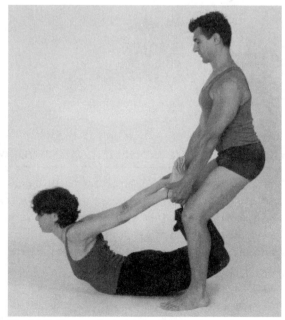

Fig. 15.3: Partner Assisted Bow Pose

on the outside of your partner's legs. Take hold of your partner's hands where they meet the ankles. Lift your partner's torso up so that his or her shoulders widen and the back lengthens (see Fig. 15.3). Hold your partner in this position for several breaths, or however long it is comfortable. To release from the pose, your partner exhales as you slowly release your hands from his or her hands and ankles. Encourage your partner to let his or her legs and feet float back down to the ground, slowly lowering the upper chest and head to the ground. Your partner rolls the head to one side and rests for several deep breaths.

Thank your partner for this opportunity to share assisted partnering, then reverse roles: You assume Bow Pose while your partner provides assisted support.

Ardha Matsyendrasana: Seated Spinal Twist

Ardha matsyendrasana, Seated Spinal Twist, is described and illustrated in Fig. YPS.10 (page 129). You can help a partner stretch even further in this position.

Have your partner sit on the floor with his or her trunk, neck, and head erect. Your partner's right leg is bent with the sole of the foot outside the straight left leg. Your partner's right arm is straight out behind him or her and the partner's left hand hugs the right knee.

Kneel behind and to the left side of your partner, facing him or her. Place your right hand on your partner's right shoulder to help it open, and place your left hand on your partner's left shoulder and encourage it to open and rotate forward. Maintain this position of support as your partner takes several deep, full breaths, opening and rotating even further to the right with each breath.

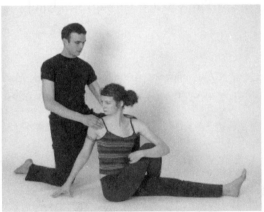

Fig. 15.4: Partner Assisted Seated Spinal Twist

Have your partner release from the pose, and then repeat Seated Spinal Twist on the other side of the body as you provide assisted support. When your partner has completed Seated Spinal Twist on both sides of the body, change roles: You assume Seated Spinal Twist successively on each side of your body while your partner assists you.

Partner Yoga: Getting Started

In Partner Yoga, you and your partner perform yoga postures together, so that you both obtain the benefits of yoga asanas at the same time. In many common Partner Yoga positions, both partners perform the same posture at the same time. Because both partners are performing yoga asanas at the same time, the positioning and body mechanics of each partner can be more complex than in Partner Assisted Yoga. For this reason, it can be helpful to do Partner Yoga under the guidance of a teacher, who can help both partners enter into the proper positions for each yoga pose.

The following postures can serve as an indication of the many yoga postures that you can enjoy with a friend, mate, or loved one in Partner Yoga.

"Double Down Dog": Partnered Downward-Facing Dog

In "Double Down Dog," both you and your partner perform Downward-Facing Dog at the same time.

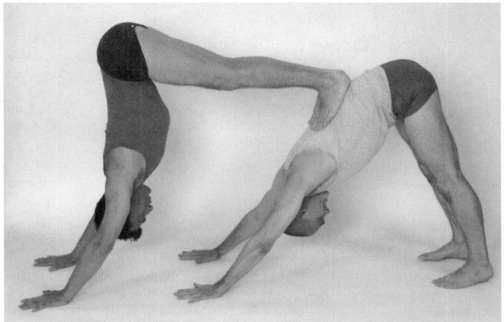

Fig. 15.5: Partner Yoga—Double Down Dog

In preparation for practicing Double Down Dog, one partner assumes Downward-Facing Dog Position (see Fig. 15.1j, page 118). The partner's feet are spread hip-width apart and the heels pressed firmly to the ground. The hands are placed shoulder-width apart. The buttocks are raised toward the ceiling so that the body forms an inverted V relative to the ground.

The second partner stands with his or her back toward the first partner. The second partner places his or her feet between the first partner's hands, and assumes Downward-Facing Dog position as previously described. The second partner bends the knees and places the hands on the floor in front, about shoulder-width apart. The second partner then raises one leg and places the foot firmly on the first partner's lower or middle back. The second partner than lifts the other foot so that it is alongside the first foot on the partner's back. The second partner straightens the arms and legs, and lifts the buttocks to assume Downward-Facing Dog position on the first partner's back (see Fig. 15.5). Hold this Double Dog Partner Yoga position for several deep breaths. The second partner then easefully returns one foot, and then the other, to the ground. Both partners can rest in Child's Pose for a few breaths, then reverse roles and perform Double Down Dog Pose once again. (**Note:** In practicing this pose, the second partner should be careful not to apply pressure directly onto the fleshly tissue just below the first partner's rib cage. If you or your partner have any back or circulatory problems, or are uncomfortable in any way, then skip this asana.)

Seated Forward Bend for Two:
Partner Yoga Seated Forward Bend

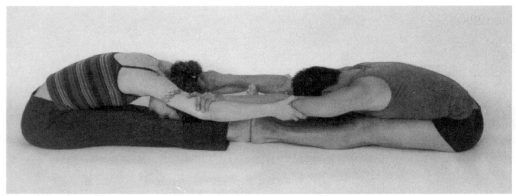

Fig. 15.6: Partner Yoga—Seated Forward Bend for Two

Performing Seated Forward Bend with a partner can help you take forward bending to new reaches. It can help you surrender to a new level of physical as well as mental and emotional release.

To perform Seated Forward Bend in Partner Yoga, both partners should sit firmly on the ground, facing one another. Legs should be straight in front of the body, with the soles of each partner's feet touching the soles of the other partner's feet. The sit-bones of both partners should be firmly rooted on the ground.

Both partners inhale as they lift the heart center and chest, raising both arms straight up overhead, parallel to one another and alongside the ears. Synchronizing the breath, both partners exhale as they reach their arms out in front of them and hold the wrists of their partner. Continuing to inhale and exhale deeply, both partners release deeper into Seated Forward Bend. The partners continue to reach so their hands move further up their partner's arms within their comfort level—holding on to the partner's elbows if possible.

Rest with your partner in Seated Forward Bend for several deep, rhythmic breaths. Synchronize your breath with your partner. As you release completely into the posture of surrender, let go of all the baggage of the past. Breathe in the present moment. Remember that you cannot breathe in the past; you cannot breathe in the future; you can only breathe in the present moment. Be totally present to yourself and your partner.

When you are both ready, each partner gently releases the arms of the other partner and inhales slowly until you are both sitting upright. Each partner should take a moment to see how he or she feels after performing Seated Forward Bend with support. Thank your partner for this opportunity to share Partner Yoga, and for supporting you in being totally present and open.

Suggested Further Resources

In this chapter, you've seen how you can incorporate yoga into your social life as well as your fitness program. If you'd like to continue to further explore yoga with a partner, the following resources are highly recommended:

Books

Cain Carroll, and Lori Kimata, N.D., *Partner Yoga: Making Contact for Physical, Emotional, and Spiritual Growth* (Rodale Press, 2000). This fully illustrated how-to book includes step-by-step directions for performing more than 60 dynamic yoga postures and three flowing yoga exercise sequences with a partner. The emphasis is on Partner Yoga rather than Partner Assisted Yoga. The authors demonstrate how two partners can perform yoga poses simultaneously, thus stretching both partners at the same time. General information on Partner Yoga is also available at the authors' Website: *www.partneryoga.com.*

Videotapes

Mark Blanchard, *Beginning Power Yoga for Couples* (Spotlight Films, 1998). In this video, Mark Blanchard and a female companion demonstrate a complete beginning Power Yoga sequence. They practice a particularly vigorous style of yoga as they alternately demonstrate on one another how one partner can assist the other in performing the poses in the sequence. Blanchard emphasizes that yoga is about union, which can mean improving your union with your partner by learning and relating to one another in new ways. While the focus is on a romantic partner, you can easily adapt the assisted postures demonstrated for use with anyone in your life—romantic or otherwise.

Living Yoga's Yoga for Two for Beginners with Rodney Yee (Living Arts, 1999). In this 20-minute instructional video, Rodney Yee and his wife, Donna Fone, demonstrate how a couple can move together to adjust one another in a gentle, flowing, synchronized yoga workout.

Kripalu Yoga Partner (Wellspring Media, 1998). The husband and wife teaching team of Todd Norian and Ann Green guide viewers through a 60-minute series of 44 "double" partnered Kripalu Yoga postures.

Websites

The Website for *Yoga Journal* contains information on a variety of yoga postures with complete instructions on how to perform each one. The description of each posture also includes information on how a partner can assist you in deepening the pose: *www.yogajournal.com.*

Cain Carroll on partner yoga for men:

"In today's fast-paced world many of us men have forgotten how to feel. Always on the run, it is easy to forget our bodies and ignore our emotions. Unfortunately, our bodies and emotions don't forget us. When ignored, tension and emotions start to pile up quickly. Our shoulders ride up to our ears, we get indigestion, feel irritated, or downright angry.

"The practice of yoga gives us an opportunity to stop and observe the situation. Through yoga we can develop sensitivity and the ability to feel body sensations and recognize emotions. This becomes an invaluable tool for maintaining radiant health. Through awareness of subtle body sensations, men learn to release tension and stress, and manage intense emotions, before they take hold and cause a problem.

"Partner Yoga gives men an opportunity to extend that awareness outward to a partner in a fun and creative way. Most partners feel that by practicing the partner poses and exercises together, they develop a better understanding of each other's bodies. Through this combined effort, each partner discovers where they store tension and how to release it. Both people feel healthier and more alive. As a result, a deeper sense of intimacy tends to emerge, and the relationship takes on a new degree of richness."

—Cain Carroll, Author of *Partner Yoga: Making Contact for Physical, Emotional, and Spiritual Growth*

PART V

THE YOGA LIFESTYLE

The focus on yoga in the West is very often placed on the physical postures of hatha yoga. This aspect of yoga appeals to many men because of the physical strength, flexibility, and grace these postures can help them achieve. Yoga can do much more than help you make the most of your body, though.

Yoga is a very rich and multifaceted web of practices. The ultimate goal of yoga is union of the individual self with the Cosmic Self. Some venerated approaches to yoga eschew the physical practices of hatha yoga in favor of other practices that foster self-reflection, such as meditation and breath awareness. Hatha yoga literally means the "forceful yoga." Some yoga sages believe that hatha yoga can be too "forceful" a path.

The *Yoga Vasistha*, one of the leading classic texts on yoga, described the experience of self-realization by a sage named Uddalaka. It recounts in detail how this man achieved bliss. Uddalaka engaged himself in austerities and the study of scriptures. He sat down in meditation and recited the sacred word Om, while he practiced special breathing techniques. And through these means, Uddalaka entered into a superconscious state in which he achieved enlightenment and liberation. It is significant that the writer of this sacred text underscores the fact that Uddalaka achieved self-realization without the practice of hatha yoga: "All this Uddalaka practiced without the violence involved in Hatha Yoga, for Hatha Yoga gives rise to pain."[1]

While the *Yoga Vasistha* describes hatha yoga as leading to pain, it certainly doesn't need to. With instruction and guidance from a qualified teacher, hatha yoga practice need not be too forceful, painful, or dangerous. Because many men think of yoga only as the practice of hatha yoga, though, it is important to know that you can also follow a path of yoga without necessarily doing the physical postures of hatha yoga. The following chapter will introduce you to additional yoga practices that you can use to round out your practice of hatha yoga or do instead of hatha yoga if you prefer.

Pursued to the fullest, yoga can help you make the most of both your body and your mind to achieve a place of inner peace and tranquility. In addition to providing guidance on beneficial physical postures, yoga can also help teach you about ways to live a healthier and more fulfilling lifestyle. If you expand your physical practice of yoga to embrace its teachings on diet, breathing exercises, and meditation, you can join the millions of other men around the world who have discovered that yoga is not only a physical discipline, but also a way of life. Chapter 16 provides valuable information on how you can make yoga a complete practice for realizing your full potential as a man.

Chapter 16

THE YOGA LIFESTYLE

Yoga as a Way of Being a Man

…The most important purpose of Yoga is to bring about a deep transformation of the individual—an awakening of intelligence that is free of dependencies and romantic beliefs and ready to meet the accelerating challenges of the 21st century.[1]

—Ganga White

The physical postures that comprise much of hatha yoga are extremely appealing to many men. They satisfy a man's need for physical exercise and provide many health benefits. They help today's overloaded man to relax, and so provide a much-sought antidote to stress. They can help a man to become more graceful, poised, and balanced in carriage and movement. They can help restore and renew both body and mind, helping men to feel clearer, lighter, and more creative. And perhaps most important of all, they can be fun and enjoyable to do in and of themselves. Because most men are first attracted to yoga for its physical health benefits, *Yoga for Men* has presented as much information as possible regarding the physical health aspects of hatha yoga to help today's man find the yoga approach that is best for him.

The ultimate goal of all yoga, including hatha yoga, however, goes beyond the physical benefits of yoga practice: It is to make the body the most perfect vehicle possible so a man can realize his total being to the fullest—body, mind, and spirit. Having a healthy and sound body is considered a prerequisite to the ability to still the mind and so achieve the higher states of concentration and meditation that lead ultimately to the realization of bliss and ecstasy as a man realizes his true nature. Hatha yoga is but one of the rungs on the ladder to self-realization.

In its largest sense, yoga is more than just the practice of physical asanas: It is a way of life—a way of being a man in the world. The eight limbs of raja yoga, discussed in Chapter 1, serve as ethical guidelines for how a man can best conduct his life so he can realize the greatest harmony both for himself and for all those around him. The teachings of yoga can serve as a much-needed roadmap to a way of life that allows men to revere the divinity in themselves and all of creation as they navigate their own unique life journeys.

The teachings of yoga are especially valuable to men at the current moment in history. According to yogic tradition, civilization undergoes extended cycles of time characterized by highs and lows, lightness and darkness. Every cycle is comprised of four stages, each of which is known as a *yuga* ("age" or "eon" in Sanskrit). These stages are very long and last for millennia. The first stage in each cycle, called a *satya yuga* ("truthful age"), is the highest point. It is characterized by prosperity, wisdom, and balance. The last stage, a *kali yuga* ("black age"), is the lowest point, and is characterized by poverty, misery, and confusion.

Yoga scholars maintain that we are currently at the beginning of a kali yuga, or a dark age. Thus, yoga theory accounts for the sense of confusion, helplessness, and aimlessness that many people today profess to experience. The events of September 11, 2001, and the ensuing chaos are but one expression of this dark undercurrent. Despite—and some might even argue because of—the rapid advances modern civilization is making in science, medicine, and technology, many people feel isolated and overwhelmed on a personal level, lacking a sense of purpose or unity in the fabric of their lives. The practice of yoga can help a man to become more centered and in touch with the essential unity of all creation.

Yoga has the powerful ability to change and transform our lives for the better. Hatha yoga has the power to begin an exciting and seemingly unending journey of self-transformation. Frequently, men who begin the practice of the physical postures of yoga merely for the physical exercise they offer find their lives changing in unexpected ways. These changes can be very subtle or more pronounced. The sense of peace and calm often engendered by the practice of yoga can help make a man more open and receptive to other changes in his life. The mindful awareness that is placed on the breath and the position of the physical body during the execution of an asana is already the beginning of a type of meditation. Men often find themselves spontaneously drawn toward meditation once they begin the physical practice of yoga. They may also change their eating habits as they gain more respect for their bodies. They may develop newfound appreciation for friends, mates, and family. They are learning firsthand that yoga is indeed more than just physical exercise: Yoga is a way of life.

Yoga has developed a variety of tools and techniques to help those who practice it progress further along their own path of self-development. These tools are wide and varied. To help you take your knowledge and practice of yoga to a further level of development should you so desire, you'll find information on the following practices in this chapter: yogic principles of diet, the science of yogic breathing (*pranayama*), and meditation. These are among the most powerful tools that yoga can offer to transform your life. I invite and encourage you to try them for yourself.

The Yogic Diet

Regulation of food is therefore the foundation of all other regulations.[2]

—Swami Rama

The yogic diet is one that takes into consideration each man's own needs as well as those of all other beings. For many yoga practitioners, this means a vegetarian diet. The practice of yoga aims to make the body a fit vehicle for universal energy, or prana, to flow through. This means that the body is much more than a machine to be nourished and maintained. It is a sacred gift. Indeed, many practitioners of yoga believe in the system of reincarnation, according to which, beings do not simply disappear upon death. Rather, the essence of each being is reincarnated in another life force—whether it is human, animal, or some other form. To be reborn as a human rather than as another object or form of being is a great gift. The gift of being human offers each man the opportunity to attain liberation through the use of his body, and just as important, his mind—the aspect of man's nature that separates him from all other beings. Therefore, men have a sacred trust to respect their bodies, as well as their minds, and so make their bodies the most fit vehicles possible to achieve enlightenment.

It is difficult indeed for a man whose body does not function well to undertake the practice of yoga. He lacks the energy to do the physical asanas or the presence and clarity of mind to engage in meditation. He lives life in a proverbial fog. The yogic approach to diet is designed to help men's bodies function as optimally as possible.

Many yogis are vegetarians because they believe that a vegetarian diet is the most healthful and energizing, and is respectful of the environment. A diet that contains meat is a much less efficient and economical diet. In order to feed the animals that we eat, many more acres full of plants are consumed than if we were to consume plants ourselves. Nearly everyone today is aware of the alarming rate at which rich natural resources such as the South American rain forests are being depleted. What many people do not know, though, is that these lands are being cleared in order to provide grazing ground for cattle and other livestock that are exported throughout the world.[3] Yogis also encourage a vegetarian diet out of respect for our fellow brethren in the animal kingdom. According to yoga philosophy, all of nature is interrelated. Through reincarnation, the animals that are alive today are just as sacred as human life. Therefore, to kill animals in order to consume them when we can survive on plants is an unnecessary harm. It violates the first of the *yamas* (or moral observances) that form the first rung of raja yoga, which is *ahimsa* (non-violence).

In addition to its recommendation of a vegetarian diet, yoga principles advise us to seek out certain foods and avoid others. In this respect, yoga is closely allied with the science of *ayurveda*, which is becoming increasingly popular in the West. Literally meaning "the science of life" in Sanskrit, ayurveda is a 5,000-year-old system of healing based on the teachings codified in the sacred Vedic literature of India. The *Vedas* ("knowledges") are the oldest recorded scriptures in India and contain much of the earliest knowledge that we have about yoga. Ayurveda uses a combination of diet, nutrition, herbs, aromatic essences, massage, crystals, visualization, and meditation, among other healing measures, to maintain and restore balance. Ayurveda, which is the oldest system of healthcare in continuous use to the present day, developed parallel to, and in tandem with, yoga. Thus, many of the principles that form the core of ayurvedic science are essential to yoga as well.

According to the wisdom that is imparted in the *Vedas*, the interplay of three primordial qualities of energy created everything that exists in the universe. These qualities of energy are called *gunas* ("strands" or "qualities"). The three gunas are *sattva, rajas*, and *tamas. Sattva* ("purity" or "virtue") represents the quality of purity. *Rajas* ("excited" or "active") represents the quality of dynamism that can be overstimulating because it assaults the system and can cause stress. *Tamas* ("darkness" or "heaviness") represents the quality of lethargy and inertia.

All foods can be grouped into three categories based on the quality of these three energies. Sattvic foods are pure foods. They are to be sought out because they can help one to achieve purity of body and mind. Sattvic foods include fruits, grains, and whole vegetables. Rajasic foods are foods that overstimulate and are to be avoided. Rajasic foods include such items as strong spices, coffee, and alcohol. Tamasic foods are foods that create lethargy and torpor, and they are to be avoided, also. Examples of tamasic foods include meat, fish, and stale and overcooked foods.[4]

In addition to following a vegetarian diet that includes sattvic foods and eschews those that are rajasic and tamasic, many adherents of yoga routinely practice ritual fasts. These fasts provide an opportunity to allow the body to eliminate toxins. Fasts can also provide a rest for the organs of digestion and other key systems in the body. Fasts are considered especially auspicious during certain days of each month, known as *ekdasi* days. Ekdasi days are 11 days after the full and new moons.[5]

Complete fasting is something that you should perform under appropriate guidance. However, many people find great benefit in undergoing limited fasts—for instance, eating only fruits for a day, or drinking juices and eating a light salad. Of course, anyone with any particular health concerns should consult a physician before undertaking the practice of fasting.

The yogic approach to diet is one that can promote health and harmony in body, mind, and spirit. To those unaccustomed to a vegetarian diet, it may seem austere. If you are interested in incorporating a yogic diet into your life, be gentle with yourself. Introduce it moderately into your life, and try not to be too hard on yourself if you cannot maintain it strictly. As with yoga, selecting the diet that is right for you can be an individual practice, and one that unfolds gradually over time.

For Further Information

If you would like to explore further how you can incorporate the yogic principle of ahimsa into your life, you may be interested in exploring vegan practices. The meanings of vegetarian and vegan (pronounced "veg-un" with a hard "g") are not the same. Vegan is a strict practice and requires the use of no animal products whatsoever in all areas of one's life—hence no products such as milk, eggs, leather, or wool. Vegetarian may include use of eggs and milk and refers only to diet. Thus a vegan is always vegetarian, but a vegetarian is not necessarily a vegan. If you are interested in learning more about vegan practices, the American Vegan Society, a nonprofit educational organization, can provide you with further information. It publishes a magazine called *American Vegan* (recently renamed from the previous title of *Ahimsa*). For further information, contact:

The American Vegan Society
56 Dinshah Lane
P.O. Box 369
Malaga, NJ
Tel: (856) 694-2887

Fax: (856) 694-2228
Website: *www.americanvegan.org*
E-mail: info@americanvegan.org

Suggested Further Reading

If you would like to experiment with a vegetarian diet, there are literally hundreds of vegetarian cookbooks available. You can visit your library or favorite bookstore and peruse the offerings to see what appeals to your sense of taste. The following are among the most popular offerings:

Deborah Madison, *Vegetarian Cooking for Everyone* (Broadway Books, 1997). The Greens restaurant in San Francisco is known for its vegetarian and vegan cuisine. In this book, the founding chef presents 1,400 recipes to appeal to both vegetarians and vegans.

The Moosewood Restaurant Cookbooks: A collective of people who rotate jobs runs The Moosewood Restaurant in Ithaca, New York, renowned for its innovative vegetarian cuisine. The Moosewood Collective has published an extensive series of cookbooks, some of them winners of the James Beard Award. The series is published by Clarkson Potter.

Pranayama: Yogic Breathing Techniques

The breath is the intelligence of the body.[6]

—T.K.V. Desikachar

Pranayama ("breath control") is the fourth limb on the eight-limbed path of raja yoga. Sometimes described as the science of breath or extension of the breath, pranayama is a highly evolved system of practices that can enable men to gain control over the breath. It follows asanas, or the practice of physical poses, on the eight-runged ladder to self-realization.

Pranayama is considered an invaluable practice because of the vital role that *prana* ("air," "breath," or "vital life-force energy") is believed to play in a man's physical, mental, and spiritual well-being. According to the tradition of yoga, prana is more than just air: It is the vital life energy that animates the being of not only every man, but also the entire world. The concept of a vital life energy that animates the entire universe is central to not only the yogic tradition, but also numerous other Asian civilizations, as well as to the belief systems of many indigenous peoples and shamanistic cultures.

Breath is life. Without oxygen, we would perish within a matter of minutes. Our first experience of life is the first breath we inhale. We intuitively know the profound wisdom of the breath. It can be an indicator of an internal, emotional state or a state of health. Shallow, rapid breathing can be a sign of internal disorder and stress. Troubled or irregular breathing can be a sign of illness. Deep, rhythmic breathing makes us feel better. When trying to calm an anxious friend, we intuitively suggest: "Take a deep breath."

Yogis have studied the power of the breath for millennia. They have discovered that by controlling the breath, we can control the mind. Thus, learning how to exercise appropriate control over the breath can be an invaluable tool on the road to liberation and the bliss of superconscious meditation.

Most people breathe in a shallow fashion—from the chest. The most efficient breathing uses the abdomen and diaphragm fully, and is often called diaphragmatic breathing. Diaphragmatic breathing is more effective than chest breathing because it allows us to take in a greater amount of oxygen. Oxygen is vital to our sustained health and well-being. Once taken into the lungs, oxygen is transferred to the blood, where it circulates throughout a man's entire system. This oxygen is transferred down to the minute cell level, where it provides the unique and essential purpose of supplying the energy that each cell needs to accomplish its role. Without oxygen, our entire system would shut down and we would die. Once oxygen has been transferred to each cell, a trade takes place whereby carbon dioxide released as a result of metabolism within each cell is exchanged back into the blood. The blood carries it to the heart and lungs, from whence it is discharged back into the atmosphere through exhalation of the breath.

This important role of oxygen is reflected in the use of the scientific term "vital capacity" to describe our ability to take in oxygen. Yogic breathing practices are designed to help us increase the amount of oxygen we take in, and consequently, increase our vital capacity.

One of the most common techniques taught in pranayama is three-part yogic breathing. This technique brings one's awareness to the breath in such a way that the duration of each inhalation and exhalation is lengthened. One does this by mindfully inhaling air in three steps: first, into the belly; next, into the mid-chest; and finally, all the way up to the shoulders and collarbones. Once the inhalation is complete, the breath is exhaled in three parts: first, from the top of the chest; second, from the mid-chest; and finally, from the abdomen. This cycle of breathing is repeated a number of times to provide increased oxygenation to the body, as well as to relax and restore.

A second popular breathing technique is called *nadi shodhanam* ("purification of the channels" or "channel cleansing"), known popularly as "Alternate Nostril Breathing." Yogis believe that energy flows through the body via a network of subtle energy channels, or nadis. Chapter 7 describes the subtle anatomy of yoga, and Fig. 7.1 (page 79) illustrates the three main energy channels that circulate through the central core. The sushumna channel runs up through the center of the spine, and the ida (associated with feminine energy) and pingala (masculine) nadis intertwine around it. Energy travels through the ida and pingala nadis in a regular, cyclic pattern. Alternate Nostril Breathing is designed to help balance the flow of masculine and feminine energy, which represent opposite poles of the self in the body. This breathing practice also helps to balance the right and left hemispheres of the brain, and has a deeply harmonizing and unifying effect on the entire body/mind/spirit.

A third common yogic breathing technique is *kapalabhati* ("lustrous") breath. It is said to be the breath that makes the entire face radiant and lustrous. This pranayama technique entails rapid, forceful exhalations of the breath and relaxed inhalations. It is said to cleanse and purify the body. In addition, it warms the body, particularly the energy in the solar plexus, which is associated with the rising of the creative kundalini energy that is believed to lie at the base of the spine. Because of its warming effect, kapalabhati breath is also popularly called "breath of fire."

There are many other yoga breathing techniques and exercises that have been developed over time. These techniques provide detailed instructions for precise ways to inhale, retain, and expel the breath. Many of these techniques are advanced and should be undertaken only under the guidance of an experienced instructor.

The three pranayama exercises described in this section, however, are simple to perform. In fact, they are often incorporated into a hatha yoga class—sometimes at the beginning or end of a class, during the performance of the physical postures themselves, or as a relaxation or energizer between postures. Because they are such powerful yoga techniques, you will find detailed information on how to incorporate them into your yoga practice in the following section. As with any technique presented in this book, however, do not undertake pranayama exercises if you have any medical concern without first consulting your primary healthcare provider.

Yogic Breathing Exercises

Yoga Breathing Exercise 1: Three-Part Yogic Breathing

Most men breathe shallowly from the chest. In three-part yogic breathing, air is inhaled into the lungs and sequentially fills the entire torso, beginning with the lower belly and rising up through the upper abdomen to chest, upper chest, and even to the shoulder area.

In preparation for doing three-part yogic breathing, it can be helpful for you to get a feeling for how you routinely breathe. To do this, lie on your back, preferably on the floor (see Fig. 16.1). Lying on a padded surface such as a rug or blanket can provide you with some cushioning. Place a pillow or bolster under your knees and/or the back of your head to increase your level of comfort in this position. You can also experiment using a rolled-up or folded towel to support your knees or head.

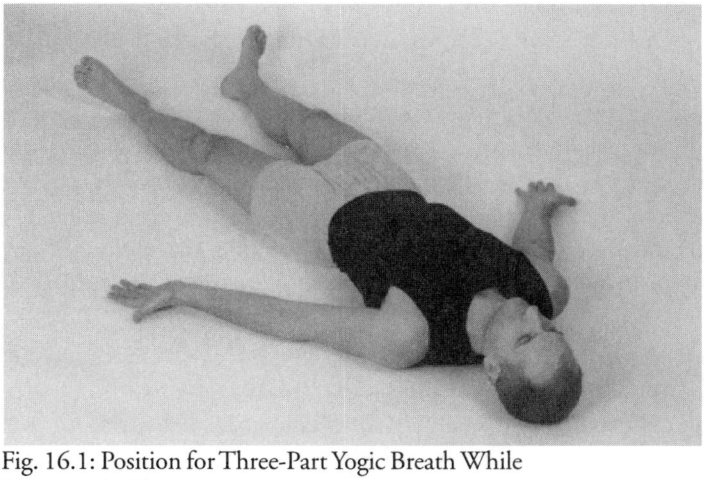

Fig. 16.1: Position for Three-Part Yogic Breath While Lying on the Floor

Breathe as you normally would: Observe your breath. If you are like most men, you are probably taking a shallow breath, mainly into the chest area. This type of breath is a shorter breath than full three-part yogic breathing, and it does not provide as rich a supply of oxygen and vital life energy as full yogic breathing.

Now, place your hands on your abdomen. As you inhale, fill up the area of your abdomen and solar plexus with as much air as you comfortably can. Do this with ease, not strain. Use your hands to feel the area of your stomach rising. Now exhale. Practice inhaling and exhaling deeply into your abdomen for several rounds of breath. You are now practicing abdominal breathing, and you are allowing your body to benefit from drawing in even more oxygen than with shallow, chest breathing.

Continue your experimentation further by placing your hands along the sides of your chest, so that your hands are covering the lateral sides of your ribs. Inhale deeply into your abdomen and allow the breath to continue to rise and fill up completely the area of your chest. With your hands, feel your ribs rising and separating as the chest fills up with rich oxygen. As you exhale, allow the breath to empty first from your chest and then from your abdomen. Feel the ribs return to their original position as the chest deflates. The abdomen also contracts. Practice several rounds of inhalation and exhalation in this manner: As you breathe in, feel your abdomen fill completely, and then your chest and ribs. As you breathe out, feel your ribs and chest deflate and your abdomen contract. Breathe slowly and rhythmically. Don't force your breath, and don't hold it, either.

Finally, to complete the introduction to three-part yogic breathing, place your hands on your upper chest, below your collarbones. As you inhale, allow your abdomen to rise as it fills with oxygen. Next, allow your chest and ribs to rise and expand. Finally, feel your upper chest, all the way out to your shoulders, expand and rise. Feel your breath rise completely with your hands resting lightly on your upper chest. As you exhale, allow the upper chest and shoulders to deflate. Allow your hands to register the sinking sensation of your upper chest as it lowers to its original position. Next, allow the air to empty out of your chest as it sinks back down. Finally, let your abdomen contract as you completely expel any remaining air. Practice breathing in and out in this fashion for several minutes: As you inhale, allow your abdomen, then chest, and finally upper chest and collarbones to fill with rich, freshly oxygenated air. As you exhale, reverse the movement: feeling your upper chest and collarbones sink back down as you breathe out, followed by the sinking of your chest, and finally, the contraction of your abdomen. You are expelling from your body all the air containing the carbon dioxide and other toxic waste products that have been created by the metabolic processes of your body's cells. You are cleansing and healing yourself all the way down to the cellular level.

After you have practiced this full three-part yogic breathing, take stock of the effects of this breathing exercise. How do you feel in relation to how you felt before you began your practice of this breathing technique? How does this type of breathing compare to your habitual way of breathing? Did any parts of this breathing have a special feeling to you— were they difficult to perform or did they feel particularly good to you? Make a note of any sensations and observations. Try not to judge yourself. Let your breath be your guide and teacher.

Practice this full three-part yogic breathing as regularly as you can. Once you are comfortable practicing it in a supine position, try practicing this yogic breathing when seated or standing. It will help you to relax and energize simultaneously. When faced with a stressful situation, taking a short break to do a few rounds of three-part yogic breathing can help calm and still your mind so that you will be better able to deal with the cares and concerns that life might throw your way.

Yoga Breathing Exercise 2: Nadi Shodhanam—Alternate Nostril Breathing

Nadi Shodhanam, or "Alternate Nostril Breathing," is a wonderful way to restore balance—physically, emotionally, and mentally. It can help to calm the nervous system, bring clarity to the mind, and may even help alleviate breathing and sinus problems.

To practice Alternate Nostril Breathing, assume a comfortable seated position. If you can, try sitting cross-legged on the floor with your sit-bones resting firmly on the ground and your trunk, spine, neck, and head erect. If this position is not comfortable for you, then try sitting in a straight-backed chair for support, with your legs uncrossed and your feet firmly resting on the ground. Let the chair or the ground support your body. In this position, also try to have your trunk, spine, neck, and head erect. A guide to the optimum posture of alignment is that a string passing through your ears, shoulders, and sit-bones would form a straight line, perpendicular to the floor. *Asana* literally means "seat." One of the key purposes of the practice of asanas, or the physical postures of hatha yoga, is to develop and maintain your body's strength and flexibility so that you can sit comfortably in an optimally aligned position for pranayama and meditation.

Allow yourself to center for a moment. Lift your right hand in front of you. Fold your index and middle fingers toward the inside of your palm. Allow your thumb and your third and little finger to remain extended outward from your right hand (see Fig. 16.2a). The position of the hand in this way forms a *mudra*, or yogic "seal" known as *mgri mudra*. *Mgri* refers to "deer" in Sanskrit: When the fingers are positioned in this way, they are said to form the shape of the antlers of a running deer when seen in profile.

Rest the back of your left hand comfortably on your left knee or thigh. Try touching the tips of the left thumb and index finger against one another, so that they form the shape of a circle. The fingers of your left hand are forming another yogic seal. This particular mudra is known as *jnana mudra*, the yogic symbol or "seal" of knowledge. Uniting the index finger and thumb represents the union of your individual consciousness with universal consciousness. This mudra helps to seal in the energy that will be circulating during your practice of Alternate Nostril Breathing.

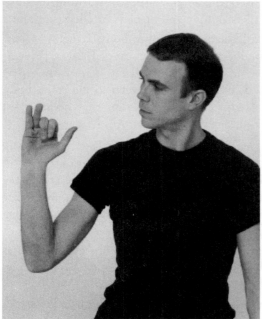

Fig. 16.2a: Alternate Nostril Breathing—Finger Positions of Right Hand

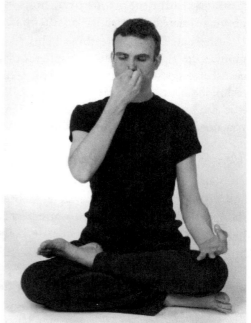

Fig. 16.2b: Alternate Nostril Breathing—Right Hand Finger Positions on Nostrils; Left Hand

Now inhale through your left nostril. As you do so, gently place your right thumb over your right nostril to seal off the nostril. You are now breathing in through the left nostril. As you complete your inhalation into your left nostril, press your right ring and little fingers gently over the left nostril as you simultaneously release your right thumb from the right nostril. Let your right thumb rest lightly on your right nostril without applying any pressure on the nostril itself so that you can exhale fully through the right nostril. You are sealing off the left nostril now as you allow your breath to release through the right nostril, thus alternating the passage of air from the left to the right nostril. On your next inhalation, maintaining the fingers of your right hand in the position where they are, inhale fully through the right nostril. As you complete your inhalation, gently release the pressure of your right ring and little fingers on the left nostril as you gently press your right thumb on your right nostril to seal it off. Exhale completely through your left nostril. You have now alternated the passage of air from the right to the left nostril. Breathing in the manner just described—in through the left nostril, out through the right; and then in through the right and out through the left—constitutes one "round" of Alternate Nostril Breathing. You begin the practice of Alternate Nostril Breathing by inhaling in through the left nostril because the left nostril represents the channel of ida, or feminine, energy in the body. As feminine energy, this channel is considered to be receptive and so is a particularly appropriate channel with which to begin to receive the intake of air in Nadi Shodhanam.

Practice as many rounds of Alternate Nostril Breathing as often as necessary until you become comfortable with it. If you are a beginner, practice three to five complete rounds of Alternate Nostril Breathing. If you are more advanced, practice 10 to 20 or more rounds. If you find that there are certain days when your sinuses are particularly congested or you have difficulty breathing through one of your nostrils, then skip the practice. You may be pleasantly surprised to discover, however, that if you do have some breathing or sinus problems, a regular practice of Alternate Nostril Breathing might help to alleviate them.

Alternate Nostril Breathing helps restore and balance the entire body. It helps to harmonize the right and left hemispheres of the brain, and the masculine and feminine energies that reside in each man. It helps to calm the nervous system, and can be just the perfect technique to use when faced with stress. Because it helps to bring oxygen to the entire body, it is also energizing. Practicing a few rounds of Alternate Nostril Breathing may be just what you need to recharge yourself during a moment of lagging energy during the day.

Yoga Breathing Exercise 3: Kapalabhati—Lustrous Breath

The yogic technique of kapalabhati, or "Lustrous Breath," is an extremely energizing and vitalizing breathing technique. It brings a great volume of oxygen into the body in a short period of time, helps to warm and invigorate the vital organs, and aids in circulating blood quickly throughout the entire body.

In preparation to practice Lustrous Breath, assume a comfortable seated position as described in "Alternate Nostril Breathing." Allow your hands to rest gently on your knee-caps, thighs, or in your lap. Take a few deep breaths to center yourself.

Now, as you breathe through your nose, contract your abdomen as you exhale. Press your navel toward your spine as you expel whatever air is in your abdomen. (See Fig. 16.3.) As soon as the air is expelled, let your abdomen relax as your body naturally inhales fresh air.

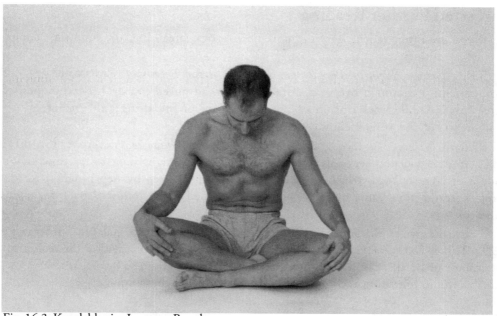

Fig. 16.3: Kapalabhati—Lustrous Breath

Then exhale once again as you contract your abdomen. Let your emphasis be on the quick, rapid, and forceful (but not forced or painful!) exhalation of air from your abdomen. Your abdomen flattens as you compress it on the exhalation, and the air naturally fills it again as you inhale. Continue exhaling and inhaling in this manner. The rapid contraction and filling of your abdomen as air is expelled and inhaled creates a type of pumping motion. If you have difficulty practicing Lustrous Breath, you might imagine that there is a feather resting on the top of your nose and you are trying to blow it off, contracting the muscles of your abdomen to initiate the exhalation. As you exhale, compress your bellybutton back toward your spine.

As you practice this breathing technique, you may want to have a handkerchief or some tissues at hand. You may find mucous secretions being more actively released from your nose on your forceful exhalations. Lustrous Breath has the added benefit of helping clear and cleanse the nasal passageways.

When you first begin to practice Lustrous Breath, try doing 20 to 30 Lustrous Breaths at a time (one active exhalation followed by a spontaneous inhalation constitutes one Lustrous Breath). Pause and rest. Then try some more. With experience, you will probably find that you can increase the period of time and numbers of inhalations and exhalations that you can accomplish without feeling fatigued.

Lustrous Breath can be particularly invigorating and energizing. As you experiment with it, see what effect it has on you. How do you feel after a round of Lustrous Breath repetitions? How do you feel relative to how you felt before you began this breathing practice? Are you aware of any difficulties or pleasurable effects that you experience as a result of this practice? As your day progresses, are you aware of any changes in your level of energy?

Suggested Further Reading

If you are interested in learning more about yogic breathing, the following books are excellent resources:

B.K.S. Iyengar, *Light on Pranayama: The Yogic Art of Breathing* (Crossroad, 1997). This book presents a thorough overview of beginning to advanced pranayama techniques, complete with a detailed description of the mechanism of breathing and extremely precise photographs of the author demonstrating each practice.

Richard Rosen, *The Yoga of Breath: A Step-by-Step Guide to Pranayama* (Shambhala, 2002). In case you find Iyengar's book too complex, you might want to try this book by a student of Iyengar Yoga, which presents a comprehensive step-by-step program for developing a steady pranayama practice, which is designed to be followed over an extended period of time.

Swami Rama, et al., *Science of Breath: A Practical Guide* (Himalayan Institute Press, 1979). This is an eminently accessible introduction to pranayama, with a discussion of the importance of breath, the mechanism of breathing, and easy-to-follow instructions on the principal yogic breathing techniques illustrated with line drawings.

Meditation

The fastest speed is not the speed of light, but the speed of mind.[7]

—Swami Rama

Many men have come to associate meditation with the practice of yoga. A common image of a yogi is that of a turbaned, revered guru sitting cross-legged in seeming meditative bliss. Maharishi Maheshi Yogi did much to popularize meditation in the West by introducing Transcendental Meditation (TM) beginning in the late 1960s through his book, *Science of Being and Art of Living: Transcendental Meditation*, and his many well-attended TM workshops. Maharishi Maheshi Yogi's TM served as the basis for Herbert Benson's groundbreaking research into the relaxation response, which further popularized meditation as an effective method of reducing stress and inducing the physiological benefits of relaxation.

Meditation now forms an integral part of many well-recognized medical programs. In his best-selling book, *The Relaxation Response*, Dr. Benson detailed many of the health benefits of meditation. Meditation helps us to enter the alpha state of brain wave activity, which is associated with relaxation and the reduction of stress. This, in turn, can help reduce blood pressure, heart rate, and speed of breathing, as well as promote healing. Meditation forms a key component of Dean Ornish, M.D.'s, celebrated program for treating heart disease. The Stress Reduction Clinic at the University of Massachusetts Medical Center bases its program for addressing stress-related disorders and chronic pain on Jon Kabat-Zinn, Ph.D.'s, mindfulness meditation training. A growing number of prestigious university training hospitals, such as Columbia-Presbyterian Medical Center in New York City, are incorporating meditation into their patient-care programs.

The words "meditation" and "medicine" are both derived from the same Latin root word. Western medical research is only now validating what practitioners of yoga have known for thousands of years: Meditation can be good medicine—a powerful tool for healing body, mind, and spirit.

One of the goals of hatha yoga is to help make the body strong, steady, and free of discomfort as a prerequisite to stilling the mind in the practice of meditation. In raja yoga, the eight-limbed path to enlightenment, *dhyana* ("meditation") is the seventh, penultimate step, preceding and leading to the state known as *samadhi* ("bliss" or "ecstasy"). Meditation is thus accorded a very important place within the practices of yoga. Contrary to a popular conception, however, meditation is not a necessary precondition to achieving enlightenment. An individual can also achieve full self-realization through other paths, such as those of karma yoga (selfless work) and bhakti yoga (unconditional devotion). (For more information on the major paths of yoga, see Chapter 1.)

Meditation can be so beneficial that it is worth exploring in greater depth. In addition to its proven benefits to physical

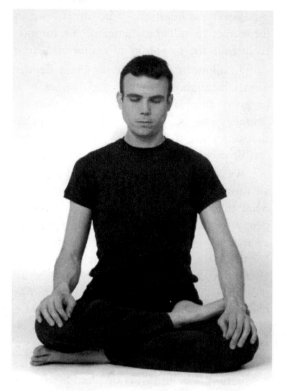

Fig. 16.4: Closed Eye Meditation Seated on the Floor

health and well-being, meditation can help a man cultivate mental and emotional stability, foster creativity, and provide a means of gaining greater insight into his higher self and purpose in life.

Meditation can be a powerful way for a man to still the mind so that he can silence for a moment the incessant chatter that occupies the rational, thinking mind. There are many ways in which to meditate, reflecting the rich diversity of meditative traditions. Each individual man's experience of meditation is unique. At heart, though, all meditative practices seek to reunite men with their deepest essence. This aim is the heart and core of yoga.

Meditation is an approach to centering oneself, of heightening one's awareness, and becoming truly present. It is not daydreaming, mindlessness, pondering weighty matters, or projecting one's fantasies. It is an opportunity simply to "be"—to realize that we are human "beings," not human "doings."

A universal concern that nags at many men, often on an unconscious level, is finding the answers to questions such as "Who am I?" and "What am I here for?" According to yogic tradition, it is necessary for a man to still the mind in order to realize his true essence. All too often, we become caught up in the affairs of the world to such an extent that they control us. We are tossed about between two extremes. We become attached to that which gives us pleasure and fear that which causes pain or discomfort. Our attachments and fears keep our minds cluttered and confused so that we are not able to go deeper into our true nature.

To answer the question "Who am I?" and so fulfill his deepest purpose in life, it is necessary for a man to still the chatter of the mind—to retreat to the realm of silence where he can truly hear the responses to important life questions emerge spontaneously.

To allow us to plumb our inner depths, yogis have developed various meditative techniques throughout the ages to help center and still the mind. By stilling the mind, we can let go of the incessant chatter that clutters what is sometimes referred to as our scattered "monkey minds." The principal method that is common to many practices of meditation is that of stilling the mind by bringing the awareness to a single object of attention. This aim can be achieved by focusing on the breath, an image, or a special sound.

Yogis know from time-honored experience that it is very difficult to empty the mind of all thoughts. It is the nature of the mind to think. Left to its natural devices, that is just what the mind will do: think incessantly. In order to help break the mind's natural tendency to chase uninterruptedly thought after thought, yogis encourage us to bring our full awareness to a single point of attention. By that means we can begin to exercise some control over the mind. By focusing on one object of attention, the meditating man, in effect, blocks out all other thoughts, thus effectively interrupting the incessant flow of thoughts. And in that moment of interruption—in the space between thoughts—a man has a window of opportunity to view and experience his true nature.

Meditation on the Breath

Meditating on the breath is one of the most basic, yet most powerful, approaches to meditation. The breath is the vital life force of the universe, and the vehicle of consciousness within us. Just sitting in quiet stillness and bringing the awareness completely to bear upon each inhalation and exhalation of the breath is one of the simplest ways of practicing meditation. As experienced meditators know, however, simple does not necessarily mean easy. It is the nature of the mind to think, so even with the clear intent to focus awareness single-pointedly upon the breath, it is the nature of the mind to wander off to pursue other thoughts. The response to this natural tendency is simply to bring the awareness gently back to the breath when such interruptions occur.

Mantra Meditation

Another popular approach to meditation is the use of a mantra. In mantra meditation, the meditator brings awareness to bear upon a special, sacred sound. The word *mantra* is derived from a Sanskrit word meaning "mind." Mantra meditation uses the power of sound to still the mind.

A mantra is a unique sound that invokes a special response. There are virtually countless mantras. Most mantras are Sanskrit words that have been passed down over the centuries by practitioners of yoga. These mantras are sounds that were determined by advanced practitioners of yoga to have special, vibratory qualities. Mystics, visionaries, and seers of ancient times discovered many of them in ecstatic states. A number of the sounds that are used as mantras refer to Hindu gods and goddesses. By repeating the sound, either out loud or mentally, the practitioner of mantra meditation experiences the quality of the divine essence with which the sound resonates. The most sacred sound of all is considered to be *Om (Aum)*, which represents the absolute. It is the most universally used mantra.

According to yogic tradition, the entire universe was created from sound. Om is the primordial sound vibration that gave rise to all of creation. Other sacred sounds include the mantra *Soham*, which in Sanskrit literally means "I am that," and so refers to one's deepest self.

Traditionally, mantras are transmitted from teacher to student by means of a rite of initiation. If you would like to try experimenting with mantra meditation, though, you could begin by using Om or Soham, as they are universally used mantras. Alternatively, you can also meditate on a word of your own choosing that has special inspirational meaning to you such as "peace" or "calm." Sometimes mantras are chanted out loud, individually or in a group. According to some yogic traditions, however, silent repetition of a mantra is even more powerful than audible repetition. Coordinating the breath with silent repetition of the mantra can make the practice of mantra recitation especially effective. For instance, a meditator could recite the sound Om silently on each inhalation and again on each exhalation of the breath. With the mantra Soham, a practitioner could silently recite the syllable "So" on each inhalation of the breath, and "ham" (pronounced "hum") on each exhalation of the breath.

Meditating on a Visual Object

Another way of focusing the awareness in meditation is to concentrate attention on a visual object. A *yantra* ("device" or "machine") is a sacred geometric representation that can be used as a device to focus visual awareness. A *mandala* is a special picture or image that can also help to concentrate awareness during meditation. The word mandala is derived from a Sanskrit word meaning "circle." Many Eastern traditions use sacred symbols as concentration devices in the practice of meditation. Mandalas often incorporate colorful and complex symbols drawn in the shape of a circle.

In addition to meditating on a special geometric symbol, you could also meditate on a picture of a sacred place; a holy person, saint, or deity; or a lighted candle. In many types of meditation, the eyes are frequently closed. However, when meditating on a visual image or object, the eyes can be left open. Eventually, adept meditators can internally visualize the object of meditation with the eyes closed. Inner visualization is considered an even more powerful form of visualization than outer visualization.

Experimenting With Meditation

The goal of hatha yoga is to prepare the body and mind for the practice of meditation. All too often, though, hatha yoga classes emphasize the practice of physical postures, with no time left for meditation at the end. If you would like to experiment with meditation, here's a basic, yet powerful, meditation you can practice on your own.

There are many ways to meditate. The following approach to meditation is probably the most universally practiced form of meditation, and among the most powerful tools for reaching that point of inner silence wherein each man can contact his highest self. Try it for yourself, either after your yoga practice, or as a separate quiet time for meditation.

Basic Closed-Eye Meditation

Find a quiet, clean, safe space for yourself. Make yourself comfortable. For greater comfort, remove your glasses and shoes if the place you are in allows you to. Assume a comfortable position, sitting on a chair, or in any cross-legged position of your choosing on the floor, spine erect but not rigid, hands softly resting on your knees or in your lap. If you are uncomfortable sitting, try lying on your back on the floor, with pillows or rolled-up towels placed under the back of your head or neck and your knees for support. (Try not to lie on a bed when you meditate because you may become so relaxed that you fall asleep!)

Close your eyes. Shrug your shoulders up toward your ears, then down toward your feet to release any tension you may be feeling.

Now bring your awareness to the point just below your nostrils. Focus on your breath. If possible, breathe in and out through your nose rather than your mouth: Breathing through the nose helps to filter, purify, and moisten the breath before it is distributed throughout the body.

On each inhalation, focus your awareness on the cool intake of air into your nostrils.

On each exhalation, feel the warm, moist outflow of breath from your nostrils.

Continue breathing in this manner for several minutes. As you inhale, be aware of the cool intake of air. As you exhale, be aware of the warm outflow of breath. Let the focus of your awareness be the breath. If your attention becomes distracted by other thoughts, just gently dismiss them and bring your awareness back to the breath.

After a few minutes, slowly bring your awareness back to your body. Feel the energy flowing to your fingers and toes. With your eyes still closed, gently stretch your fingers and toes. Rub your hands together and cup the palms lightly over your eyes. Feel the warmth of your hands restoring and energizing you. When you are ready, slowly open your eyes. Keep your hands cupped over your eyes for a moment while you adjust to the light, and then slowly release your hands. Take a moment to notice any changes in how you feel or how you perceive your surroundings.

This basic meditation can help to make you feel more relaxed and centered. It can give you renewed energy and help you to think more clearly. It can be used to start your day, as a stress-buster during a busy day of work, or as a way of clearing mental debris at the end of a workday. The greatest benefits of meditation will come with regular practice. Through meditation, the mind can become more centered and clear. This provides an ideal opportunity for you to access your deepest, inherent wisdom.

As you deepen your practice of meditation, try extending your period of meditation in small increments until gradually you are meditating for a period of 15 minutes. Try meditating early in the morning if you can, after you've gotten up and done your morning ritual, and before starting the workday. As you progress, you might also add a 15-minute period of meditation at the end of the workday to clear your mind of the clutter of thoughts and feelings that have accumulated during the morning and afternoon, and so restore yourself as you prepare for your evening activities. You can experiment with meditating before going to sleep. Be aware, though, that some people get a burst of energy either immediately following or several hours after meditating, so it might interfere with your sleep. Try not to meditate as you're lying in bed trying to fall asleep because you may begin to equate meditation with sleep, and the two are different processes. Early morning and early evening seem to be especially auspicious times for meditation. This is echoed in many diverse religious traditions, which place the time for recitation of sacred prayers at dawn and dusk.

If you would like to try meditating with a mantra or a visual image, you can follow the guidelines for the basic meditation, using a sound, word, or image as your object of concentration. Whatever the method of meditation you practice, allow your breath to be as full, natural, and deep as possible.

You might also practice meditation while walking or going about daily activities, in a practice sometimes referred to as "mindfulness" meditation. Remember: If you focus on your breath as you sit, lie, walk, or move about, it will always bring you back to awareness of the present moment. We cannot breathe in the past; we cannot breathe in the future; we can only breathe in the present. Breath is life itself; it is the gateway to our inner being. If you follow your breath with consciousness, the breath can be your best guide to your deepest self.

For Further Information

If you'd like to take a meditation course, you'll find opportunities available in nearly any city or town to do so. Many community groups, learning centers, yoga groups, and even the local YMCA or YMHA offer introductory courses. Also, check announcements on the bulletin board of your local health-food store for classes that may be offered in your area. Virtually all of the yoga organizations and institutes listed throughout this book either offer courses in meditation or can help you find a resource near you.

Suggested Further Resources

There are literally hundreds, if not thousands, of books, audiotapes, videos, and even CD-ROMs and DVDs on meditation. Just a few of the most well-known presenters on the subject include Ram Dass, Jack Kornfield, Stephen Levine, Shunryu Suzuki, and Thich Nhat Hanh. Their books and tapes are widely available. In addition, many organizations, including those cited throughout *Yoga for Men*, publish or distribute a range of materials related to meditation.

Go to your local library or bookstore and explore its selection of books on meditation. Let your inner wisdom guide you to the resources that speak to your deepest self.

Swami Sivananda on the yoga way of life:

"Get up at 4 a.m. daily. Do Japa (mantra recitation) and meditation.

Take Sattwic (pure) Ahara (food). Do not overload the stomach.

Sit in Padma (lotus) or Siddha (perfect) asana for Japa and Dhyana (meditation).

Have a separate meditation room under lock and key.

Do charity one tenth of your income.

Study systematically one chapter *Bhagavad Gita.*

Preserve Veerya (the vital force). Sleep separately.

Give up smoking, intoxicating drinks, and rajasic (stimulating) food.

Fast on Ekdashi (auspicious fasting) days or live on milk and fruits only.

Observe Mowna (silence) for two hours daily and during meals also.

Speak Trush at any cost. Speak a little.

Reduce your wants. Lead a happy, contented life.

Never hurt the feelings of others. Be kind to all.

Think of the mistakes you have done (self-analysis).

Do not depend on servants. Have self-reliance.

Think of God as soon as you get up and when you go to bed.

Have always a Japa Mala (rosary) around your neck or in your pocket.

Have the motto: "Simple living and high thinking."

Serve Sadhus, Sannyasins (virtuous people) and poor and sick persons.

Keep a daily spiritual diary. Stick to your routine."[8]

—Swami Sivananda's *Twenty Spiritual Instructions*

Mark Donato on yoga, breath, and "being":

"When I was a boy, my family thought I had a hearing problem. What was happening was that I was deeply caught up in my creative imagination—thinking of unicorns, dolphins, and performing in movie musicals. I wasn't being present to the moment, and so I didn't hear them.

"For years, my family kept insisting that I had this hearing problem. This got very annoying because I knew that my hearing was fine. Eventually, my parents had my hearing checked by a doctor. The doctor confirmed that there were no problems.

"The sitting meditation practice I now teach has us watching our breath as a way of being in the present moment. When thoughts pop up in our heads, we label them 'thinking,' exhale, and come back to our breath. Thoughts are about the past or the future. Being in the present moment is a state of being, not of thinking.

"Now, having a creative imagination is a good thing. But yoga teaches us to be creative yet remain present at the same time. We synchronize breath and movement to balance body and mind."

—Mark Donato, a boy who grew up to be a performing artist and yoga teacher

PART VI

SUPPLEMENTAL RESOURCE
INFORMATION

In this section, you'll find helpful information to supplement your knowledge of the rich and varied world of yoga.

Chapter 17

RESOURCES FOR FURTHER EXPLORATION

Yoga Classes: Finding a Class Near You

One of the best ways to explore yoga is to take a class. Nothing beats the expert guidance and support of an experienced teacher. Yoga has become so popular that it should be easy to find a class in your area, whether you live in a major urban center or in a more remote city or town. Many health clubs now offer yoga classes as part of their overall fitness programs. Other good places to check are your local YMCA or YMHA and your town's community center.

You can check for yoga classes in the yellow pages of your local telephone directory (usually listed under "Yoga"). You can also explore the bulletin boards of local health-food stores, massage therapy offices, and metaphysical bookstores—often, teachers of yoga post announcements about classes they offer at such sites. Your local adult education or learning exchange might also offer courses in yoga.

Finally, you can check with the national associations of the major yoga institutes and associations. Often, they maintain databases of certified yoga teachers that are available in your area. You can do much of your research on the Internet if you choose, as virtually every major institute and association now has a Website with helpful information, which often includes a searchable listing of teachers by state, city, and even zip code, as well as valuable links to other yoga resources. At the end of this chapter you will find sections on "Yoga Resources on the Internet," which may be of additional assistance to you.

When evaluating a potential yoga teacher, try to find out what the background and experience of the yoga teacher is, as well as what particular style or styles of yoga the teacher incorporates into the classes. It is becoming increasingly more common for yoga teachers to study more than one approach to yoga as they deepen their own practice. If a prospective teacher blends several styles together, ask what styles are being used. For further tips on choosing a yoga teacher and preparing for your yoga class, please see "Helpful Hints" on page 19.

Yoga Courses, Workshops, and Retreats

One excellent way to explore yoga is to enroll in a short course or workshop in yoga. This way, you can begin or strengthen your yoga practice by working in an extended fashion under competent supervision. Many of the institutes representing major styles of yoga, such as the Himalayan Institute, Integral Yoga, Iyengar Yoga, and Sivananda Yoga offer series of courses in yoga, graded to different levels of practitioners (for instance, Beginners, Intermediate, and Advanced practitioners). Many yoga institutes and studios also offer intensive workshops in a particular aspect of yoga practice, such as a weekend afternoon workshop on how to achieve the perfect headstand.

Another way to immerse yourself intensively in yoga is to attend a yoga workshop or retreat that spans several days. If you attend a retreat in a picturesque setting, you can combine your practice of yoga with a bit of vacation spent in the company of other individuals who perhaps share interests similar to your own. If you travel to a more distant location, your experience can be even more exotic and mind-expanding.

Many of the yoga institutes and associations listed throughout *Yoga for Men* offer workshops and retreats. If you are interested in experiencing a particular style of yoga, check with an association that is affiliated with that style. In addition to the major yoga associations, the following organizations offer workshops and retreats in yoga:

Elat Chayyim offers courses in meditation and yoga within a Jewish spiritual environment. Recent representative samplings of retreat courses offered include "Torah Yoga for Healing and Transformation" and "Yoga and Meditation: Breathing into Balance." Of special interest to readers of *Yoga for Men*, it offers programs such as "Jewish Men's Retreat."

Elat Chayyim
99 Mill Hook Road
Accord, NY 12404
Tel: (800) 398-2630 or (845) 626-0157
Fax: (845) 626-2037
Website: *www.elatchayyim.org*
E-mail: info@elatchayyim.org

Esalen Institute is one of the premier learning centers in the United States, and a pioneer in the human potential movement. It offers a wide variety of courses and workshops in yoga—representative programs include Hatha Yoga, Nada Yoga (the yoga of sound), Vinyasa Yoga and Trance Dance, Chakra Integration, Yoga in Action, and a Labor-of-Love Yoga Retreat weekend. In addition, Esalen offers a month-long yoga work/study program for individuals who want an in-depth immersion. For the man who wishes to pamper himself, Esalen boasts hot springs and a variety of bodywork treatments in many different styles.

Esalen Institute
55000 Highway 1
Big Sur, CA 93920-9616
Tel: (831) 667-3000 (general information) or (408) 667-3005 (reservations only)
Fax: (831) 667-2724 (exclusively for reservations; no general correspondence)
Website: *www.esalen.org*
E-mail: info@esalen.org

The Expanding Light Retreat offers programs year-round in yoga, meditation, and healthy lifestyle education. The keystone of The Expanding Light's approach to yoga is Ananda Yoga for Higher Awareness. (For more information on this approach to yoga, please see the entry on "Ananda Yoga," page 99.)

The Expanding Light Retreat
14618 Tyler Foote Road
Nevada City, CA 95959
Tel: (800) 346-5350 or (530) 478-7518
Fax: (530) 478-7518
Website: *www.expandinglight.org*
E-mail: info@expandinglight.org

The Feathered Pipe Foundation offers week-long yoga workshops with some of the best-known teachers of yoga in the United States at several locations, including the Feathered Pipe Ranch, a quiet pristine wilderness retreat center in the Montana Rockies, and other interesting and exotic locations, such as Bhutan and Mexico.

Feathered Pipe Ranch
The Feathered Pipe Foundation
P.O. Box 1682
Helena, MT 59624
Voicemail: (406) 442-8196
Fax: (406) 442-8110
Website: *www.featheredpipe.com*
E-mail: fpranch@mt.net

The Himalayan Institute offers a wide variety of programs on yoga and healthy living both at its main headquarters in Honesdale, Pennsylvania, as well as at its numerous branch locations throughout the United States and the rest of the world. For more information on the Institute and its tradition of yoga, see Chapter 2. Of interest to those men wishing to immerse themselves more fully in the yoga lifestyle, the Institute offers residential programs ranging from days to months at its Honesdale campus. Its Self-Transformation Program, ranging from one to three months, provides a complete introduction to yoga practices by taking part in a variety of courses and seminars offered throughout the week and on weekends. Participants in the program perform four to five hours of selfless community service from Monday to Saturday to contribute to community life through work. This allows them to put into practice the teachings and practice of yoga in daily living activities.

Himalayan Institute
RR1 Box 1127
Honesdale, PA 18431-9706
Tel: (800) 822-4547 or (570) 253-5551
Fax: (570) 253-9078
Website: *www.himalayaninstitute.org*
E-mail: info@himalayaninstitute.org

Hollyhock Retreat Center, which recently celebrated its 20th anniversary, is Canada's leading education retreat and an international center for the cultivation of human consciousness, well-being, and social impact. It is located on the spectacularly scenic Cortes Island, off the western coast of Canada. To the man seeking an active vacation/retreat experience, it offers such diverse possibilities as hiking, swimming, sailing, and kayaking. It offers a wide range of courses and workshops in yoga. Recent offerings include programs in Ashtanga Yoga, Iyengar Yoga, karma yoga, and Kripalu Yoga, among others. As a sign of the popularity of the yoga practiced at Hollyhock, one recent work/study program called "Yoga and the Expressive Arts" was sold-out well in advance of its start date.

Hollyhock Retreat Center
P.O. Box 127
Manson's Landing
Cortes Landing, B.C.
Canada V0P 1K0
Tel: (800) 933-6339 or (250) 935-6576 (outside North America)
Fax: (250) 935-6424
Website: *www.hollyhock.ca*
E-mail: registration@hollyhock.ca

Kripalu Center for Yoga and Health is a holistic center located in the scenic Berkshire Mountains. In addition to offering classes and teacher training certification in its own approach to yoga (see Chapter 8), it offers weekend retreats as well as intensive yoga conferences that bring together some of the foremost yoga teachers in the world. In addition, for the man seeking a deeper immersion into yoga while taking some time away from the workaday world, Kripalu offers a three-month intensive Spiritual Lifestyle Program (SLP). The program is designed for people who are ready to make a deep commitment to transformation at all levels—physical, emotional, mental, and spiritual. The essence of SLP is karma yoga, learning to use work as a spiritual practice. SLP participants serve 40 hours per week, generally making beds, washing dishes, and cleaning. They also receive general training in yogic living, including hatha yoga classes, study groups, and sharing groups designed to deepen and support their SLP experience. SLP is a work exchange program that does not require a fee.

Kripalu Center for Yoga and Health

Box 793

Lenox, MA 01240

Tel: (800) 741-SELF (7353) or (413) 448-3152 (international and local calls)

Fax: (413) 448-3384

Website: *www.kripalu.org*

E-mail: request@kripalu.org (for general questions or to request a catalog)

The Mount Madonna Center is inspired by Baba Hari Dass and is sponsored by the Hanuman Fellowship, a group whose talents and interests are unified by the common practice of yoga. Located south of San Francisco between Watsonville and Gilroy, the Center offers a wide variety of courses and programs in yoga. Mount Madonna Center occupies 355 acres overlooking all of Monterey Bay. Amenities that may appeal to the active man include hiking trails, volleyball, tennis, and basketball courts, a small lake for swimming, a hot tub, and a gymnasium for volleyball and basketball. Accommodations range from campgrounds to private rooms with baths.

Mount Madonna Center

445 Summit Road

Watsonville, CA 95076

Tel: (408) 847-0406

Fax: (408) 847-2683

Website: *www.mountmadonna.org*

E-mail: programs@mountmadonna.org

Omega Institute for Holistic Studies offers some of the most broad-based and widely available holistic courses and programs in the United States. Headquartered in Rhinebeck, New York, it offers programs in an array of yoga styles, as well as yoga teacher certification programs. It presents workshops during the winter at such warm holiday destinations as the Caribbean (St. John, U.S. Virgin Islands) and Costa Rica. During the year, it offers weekend conferences and one-day courses at major urban areas and retreat centers throughout the country, including Austin, Boston, Miami, and New York City. Of special interest to yoga devotees is its Annual Yoga Conference, which brings together some of the best-known teachers of yoga for several days of intense lectures and workshops.

Omega Institute for Holistic Studies

150 Lake Drive

Rhinebeck, NY 12572

Tel: (845) 266-4444 or (800) 944-1001 (registration)

Fax: (845) 266-3679

Website: *www.eomega.org*

E-mail: registration@eomega.org

Resources for Further Reading

Periodicals

The following periodicals are either devoted to the practice of yoga or frequently contain articles of interest related to the subject of yoga:

Body & Soul Magazine is a bimonthly publication that features articles on subjects that help nourish body and soul, including yoga and related topics. For further information contact:

New Age Publishing

42 Pleasant Street

Watertown, MA 02472

Tel: (617) 926-0200

Fax: (617) 926-5021

Website: *www.bodyandsoulmag.com*

Yoga International is published bimonthly by the Himalayan Institute, a nonprofit organization. The mission of this periodical is to promote world peace through nonviolence, the harmony of existing faiths and religions, and self-discipline for individual growth on three levels: spiritual, mental, and physical. In addition to its ongoing magazine, the Himlayan Institute's Website contains valuable information regarding up-to-date information on yoga teachers, training programs, and associations throughout the United States. It also includes a rich archive of articles on yoga. For further information contact:

Himalayan Institute of Yoga Science and Philosophy of the USA

RR 1 Box 1127

Honesdale, PA 18431-9706

Tel: (800) 822-4547 or (570) 253-5551

Fax: (570) 253-9078

Website: *www.himalayaninstitue.org*

E-mail: info@himalayaninstitute.org

Yoga Journal is published bimonthly. Founded in 1975 by the California Yoga Teachers Association, a nonprofit educational corporation, it is now privately held and produced. For more than 25 years, it has published a wide-ranging collection of articles on yoga and yoga-related topics. For further information contact:

Yoga Journal

2054 University Avenue

Berkeley, CA 94704-1082

Tel: (510) 841-9200 (9 a.m. to 5 p.m. Pacific Standard Time)

Fax: (510) 644-3101

Website: *www.yogajournal.com*

For subscriptions contact:

Yoga Journal

P.O. Box 469018

Escondido, CA 92046-9018

Tel: (800) 334-8152

E-mail: yogajournal@neodata.com

Men's Health is a magazine devoted to, and regularly publishes information on, issues of men's health and fitness, including yoga. It also has a Website, where you'll find a wealth of information online:

Men's Health magazine

Rodale Inc.

33 East Minor Street

Emmaus, PA 18098-0099

Tel: (800) 666-2303 (Subscriptions)

Tel: (610) 967-5171 (Rodale Press)

Fax: (610) 967-7725 (*Men's Health* magazine)

Website: *www.menshealth.com*

E-mail: MensHealth@Rodale.com

Mail-Order Book Companies

If you're interested in pursuing any of the suggested further reading in this book, the following mail-order book companies have a wide selection of books on yoga and complementary wellness and self-care practices. Details of many of the books they carry are available on the Internet via their Websites and by mail by periodically printed catalogs.

East West Books

(Affiliated with the Himalayan Institute)

78 Fifth Avenue

New York, NY 10011

Tel: (877) 742-6844 or (212) 243-5994

For information on East West Books, please visit the Himalayan Institute Website at: *www.himalayaninstitute.org*.

East West Bookshop

(Affiliated with Ananda/The Expanding Light)

324 Castro Street

Mountain View, CA 94041-1297

Tel: (800) 909-6161 or (650) 988-9800

Website: *www.eastwest.com*

E-mail: info@eastwest.com

Integral Yoga Distribution

Satchidananda Ashram-Yogaville

Route 1, Box 1720

Buckingham, VA 23921

Tel: (800) 262-1008 or (434) 969-1040 (local calls)

Website: *www.yogahealthbooks.com*

Redwing Reviews

44 Linden Street

Brookline, MA 02445

Tel: (800) 873-3946 (toll-free United States), (888) 873-3947 (toll-free Canada), or (617) 738-4664 (worldwide)

Fax: (617) 738-4620

Website: *www.redwingbooks.com*

E-mail: info@redwingbooks.com (general information)

Book Publishers

While many fine publishing companies, including large commercial publishers, present books on yoga, the following smaller presses regularly publish books of interest on yoga and issues related to men's health:

Career Press/New Page Books

3 Tice Road, P.O. Box 687

Franklin Lakes, NJ 07417

Tel: (800) 227-3371or (201) 848-0310 (New Jersey only)

Website: *www.newpagebooks.com*

E-mail: bbrienza@newpagebooks.com

Inner Traditions * Bear and Company

One Park Street

Rochester, VT 05767

Tel: (800) 340-2432 (orders) or (802) 767-3174 (publisher)

Fax: (802) 767-3728

Website: *www.InnerTraditions.com*

E-mail: info@InnerTraditions.com

Rodmell Press

2147 Blake Street

Berkeley, CA 94704-2715

Tel: (510) 841-3123

Fax: (510) 841-3191

Website: *www.rodmellpress.com*

E-mail: info@rodmellpress.com

Rudra Press
P.O. Box 13310
Portland, OR 97213-0390
Tel: (800) 876-7798
Fax: (503) 236-9878
Website: *www.rudrapress.com*
E-mail: rudra@rudrapress.com

Shambhala Publications, Inc.
Horticultural Hall
300 Massachusetts Avenue
Boston, MA 02115
Tel: (866) 424-0030 (customer service)
Fax: (617) 236-1563
Website: *www.shambhala.com*
E-mail: editors@shambhala.com

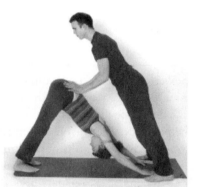

A yoga sticky mat can help prevent sliding while doing yoga.

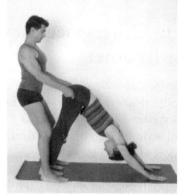

A yoga belt or strap can help provide added support and assistance in various poses.

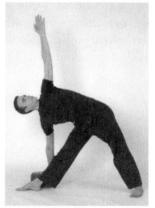

A yoga block can help provide support and stability in standing poses.

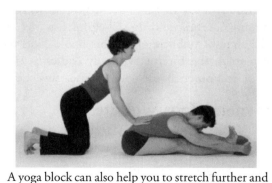

A yoga block can also help you to stretch further and longer.

Yoga Accessories and Props

When practicing yoga, it can be helpful to incorporate the use of an assortment of accessories designed to enhance your practice and make it as rewarding as possible. Such accessories, or props, include sticky mats, yoga belts, wood and foam blocks, and a variety of devices specially designed to support you in performing a variety of postures. The following companies stock a wide selection of yoga accessories as well as books, videos, and audio recordings to enhance your yoga practice. Information for all these companies' products can be obtained online:

Bheka Yoga Supplies: *www.bheka.com*

Gaiam/Living Arts: *www.gaiam.com*

Half Moon Yoga Props: *www.halfmoonyogaprops.com*

Hugger-Mugger Yoga Products: *www.huggermugger.com*

Tools for Yoga: *www.toolsforyoga.net*

Yoga Pro: *www.yogapro.com*

Yoga Props: *www.yogaprops.net*

Yoga in Cyberspace: Resources for Yoga on the Internet

As many men are discovering, the Internet is a powerful resource that connects you to a vast body of information quickly. Due to the increasing popularity of yoga, the number of Websites devoted to this subject is growing at a rapid rate. Virtually every major school or organized style of yoga has a Website that provides helpful information on its approach to yoga, valuable information on yoga in general, and, frequently, links to other helpful sites. The most recently available information on these Internet sites is included in the chapters on individual styles of yoga. In addition, the Websites for any learning networks that are cited in this chapter are included with their descriptive entries.

In addition to the information available from the yoga institutes and learning networks featured so far in this book, the following is a list of some additional Websites that are among the best and most helpful Internet sites regarding yoga and men's health issues at the time of publication of this book. Sites frequently have links to other related sites: You can roam the Internet virtually endlessly, finding more and more about yoga. So turn on your computer, point your mouse, and start surfing!

General Yoga Websites

American Institute of Vedic Studies: *www.vedanet.com*

Founded by Dr. David Frawley (Pandit Vamadeva Shastri), the American Institute of Vedic Studies is an educational and research center devoted to the greater system of Vedic and yogic knowledge, including ayurveda, vedic astrology, yoga, tantra, and vedanta.

Capeller's Sanskrit-English Dictionary: *www.uni-koeln.de/phil-fak/indologie/tamil/ cap_search.html*

Capeller's Sanskrit-English Dictionary is part of the Cologne Digital Sanskrit Dictionary project. If you are interested in exploring more about the Sanskrit terms that are used in yoga, it is a wonderful source of information. It was invaluable in verifying translations when writing this book.

Natural Health magazine online: *www.naturalhealth1.com*

Natural Health (formerly *East/West*) is dedicated to promoting well-being through approaches that nurture self-healing. While not a yoga-specific Website, it has articles and columns on yoga and related topics such as health and fitness.

Yoga.com: *www.yoga.com*

Yoga.com was developed with the mission of presenting helpful information, including the latest trends in yoga, wellness, and fitness. It includes much useful information on yoga, including a library of articles.

Yoga Alliance: *www.yogaalliance.org*

The Yoga Alliance is the first and (at the time of the writing of this book) only national organization providing a registry of yoga teachers and yoga schools that meet specific minimum standards of training.

Yoga International magazine: *www.yimag.org*

This is the Website of *Yoga International* magazine. It contains a wealth of information, including archived articles on yoga.

Yoga Journal: *www.yogajournal.com*

This is the Website of *Yoga Journal*. It is also a rich source of information, including archived articles on yoga.

Yoga Online: *indigo.ie/~cmouze/yoga_online/links.htm*

This rather cumbersome URL address is the "links" page of Yoga Online. It is a directory of yoga resources on the Internet. It can help provide you with a link to numerous yoga organizations and associations.

Yoga Research Education Center: *www.yrec.org*

This is the home page of the Yoga Research and Education Center (YREC). The YREC is a nonprofit organization founded by Georg Feuerstein, one of the leading authorities on yoga. It offers spiritual practitioners and students of yoga a wide variety of offerings, including articles and information on the history, philosophy, and practice of yoga and the spiritual traditions associated with the practice of yoga. The Website content is updated with current articles and links to other yoga-related Websites. Georg Feuerstein has made a priceless contribution to the understanding of yoga through the many books that he has authored. His writings have helped me personally to deepen my understanding of yoga over the years, and have served as reference points for verifying the accuracy of some of the information contained in this book. On this Website, he shares much of his vast knowledge of yoga.

International Association of Yoga Therapists: *www.iayt.org*

The International Association of Yoga Therapists is a division of the YREC that champions the cause of yoga and serves teachers of yoga—particularly those who use it therapeutically. This Website is a truly wonderful resource.

Yogafinder.com: *www.yogafinder.com*

Yogafinder.com bills itself as the largest yoga directory on the Internet, with information on yoga classes, teacher training, retreats, and yoga products. Of special note, it allows you to search by state and city for a teacher of a particular style of yoga. So if you've found an approach to yoga in *Yoga for Men* that you'd like to try, you might use this site to see where the closest teacher of that approach is located.

Websites With Information on Yoga for Men and Men's Health and Fitness

AskMen: *www.AskMen.com*

This is a searchable database in which you can type in a subject (such as yoga) and quickly find a number of articles and links to help answer your questions.

Gaysports: *www.gaysports.com*

While this site is targeted to a gay audience, it contains a host of information on male fitness including yoga that can be helpful to any man.

Guyville: *www.guyville.com*

This is a Website full of information on many subjects, including health and fitness, for every guy.

Men's Fitness Magazine: *www.mensfitness.com*

This is the Website of *Men's Fitness* magazine, which contains articles on topics related to men's health and fitness.

Malehealthcenter: *www.malehealthcenter.com*

This is the Website of the Male Health Center, located in Denver, Colorado, and the first health center in the United States to be dedicated to the issue of men's health.

Menstuff: *www.menstuff.org*

This Website has compiled information and books on the issue of yoga for men, as well as other topics relevant to men's health and fitness.

PROACT (Prostate Action, Inc.): *www.prostateaction.org*

PROACT (Prostate Action, Inc.) is a nonprofit organization with a mission to help men make informed decisions about preserving and protecting their health by promoting greater public awareness of and understanding about prostate diseases. It was founded in 1994 by William C. Roher, a prostate cancer survivor.

Prostate Cancer Educational Council (PCEC): *www.pcaw.com*

The Prostate Cancer Educational Council (PCEC) is a nonprofit organization that founded and coordinates the National Cancer Prostate Cancer Awareness Week Program. Its Website is a rich source of articles on prostate disease, with links to other useful resources.

Prostate Forum: *www.prostateforum.com*

The *Prostate Forum* is a subscription-based monthly newsletter created in 1996 by Dr. Charles Myers, a leader in prostate cancer treatment and research, and his wife, Rose Sgarlat Myers. The purpose of the newsletter is to provide useful, reliable, timely information about prostate cancer and its treatment in easy-to-understand language.

The Web and You

The Web is a powerful tool for researching information that best suits your needs and interests. So if you have access to the Internet, become a cybernaut. Use popular search tools, such as Google, Lycos, Yahoo, your Internet service provider, or your own preferred search engine to fine-tune your investigation of yoga. Type in the keywords regarding yoga that most interest you, click your mouse, and learn. When surfing the Web, be aware that the content of many Websites has not been subject to outside, objective verification. Use your own judgment to evaluate the reliability and pertinence of what you find.

As you sit at your computer, think about taking a periodic yoga break. Try doing some yoga stretches to relieve any stiffness you may get from sitting in a fixed position for a period of time.

And remember, as with all you do with yoga, have fun!

THE YOGA PUZZLE

Putting the Pieces Together

Our body is a friend that will rarely let us down, anytime we want to find the way "home."[1]

—Michael Lee

The Yoga Puzzle

For today's man, the world of yoga offers a rich and varied menu of principles and styles of yoga practice from which to choose. It is for this reason that *Yoga for Men* has presented information on a wide range of commonly available approaches to yoga so that you might make the most informed decision possible about what style of yoga might be right for you. Only a few years ago, you might only have had the option of taking a class labeled generically as "hatha yoga" at your local yoga studio or health club. Today, you can choose from Ashtanga, Bikram, Kundalini, Phoenix Rising, Sivananda, and scores of other approaches. You can also choose to incorporate yogic principles of diet, meditation, and breathing practices into your lifestyle. It's no wonder that even seasoned yogis are sometimes confused about how yoga might best satisfy their current needs.

The world of yoga today may seem like a puzzle to some men. With so many pieces scattered about, how do you put them together to custom-tailor the yoga practice that's just right for you? To choose the yoga way that's right for you, you might want to consider some of the general guidelines given below as you piece your yoga program together.[2]

Piece #1: Define the Overall Goals of Your Yoga Practice

In selecting the yoga style or styles that will help you most, take the time to consider first what you are looking for in your yoga practice. Are you looking for an intense physical workout? Are you looking for a relaxing yoga practice that will help you de-stress while strengthening and toning your body? Are you more interested in pursuing yoga's therapeutic benefits—either from a physical point of view in terms of dealing with particular physical challenges or issues—or from an emotional and psychological point of view in terms of helping to get clarity on deeper core issues?

Are you a perfectionist who is looking for guidance in how to attain and hold the "perfect" yoga posture? Are you more interested in yoga as an entire lifestyle, seeking direction in diet and instruction in meditation, or benefiting from yogic breathing techniques? Are you perhaps more of a spiritual aspirant, not so concerned with the physical exercises of yoga, but looking to penetrate the deep wisdom of the spiritual tradition of yoga?

Understanding what you are hoping to gain from yoga can help you custom-tailor a yoga practice that's right for you—taking into account your individual needs at this moment in time. In this way, you can creatively join the pieces of yoga that will be most appropriate for you.

Of course, as with many men, you may have more than one goal in mind when practicing yoga. You may want an intense physical workout, while at the same time hoping for some relaxation and peace of mind, or maybe even a glimmer or more of spiritual enlightenment. Your needs may change from day to day—perhaps one day you want a vigorous workout and the next day you want to practice yoga in a way that's physically less demanding.

A good yoga teacher in nearly any style of yoga should be able to help you develop a yoga program that will suit your needs. In addition, as you gain experience in your practice of yoga, you will become your own teacher. The mindfulness of yoga will most likely help you to become more in tune with your own body. You'll learn to know what you and your body/mind/spirit need most at any given moment. In that way, you'll be able to modify your yoga practice to suit your needs. If you feel like you need a vigorous workout, you can go all out in your hatha yoga practice. If you feel like your body needs to rest a bit, you can perform your yoga practice in a gentler way: Even in a vigorous style of yoga, you can practice in a softer and gentler way. And in any yoga practice or class, you can always just stop altogether to relax in Child's Pose or Corpse Pose (Fig. YPS.2a, b, and YPS.3 on pages 121–122) to allow your body to restore and renew. By learning to listen to your body and its needs, with time you will become your own best yoga teacher.

Piece #2: Realistically Assess Your Current Overall Fitness Level

In determining the yoga practice that's right for you, it's also important that you realistically assess your current overall general fitness condition—and that includes your states of physical, emotional, and mental health. You may have the desire to begin a practice of vigorous athletic-style yoga, but if you have been a couch potato for years and are in poor physical training, you might more realistically begin with a gentler style of yoga and work up gradually to a more difficult practice. You may want to open the floodways of kundalini energy in your body, but if you are going through a period of difficult emotional or mental trauma, a practice of kundalini yoga (see Chapter 7) might aggravate, rather than help, your situation. So in deciding how to tailor your own individual yoga program, be aware not only of your ideals in practice, but also your realistic starting point.

Having taken stock of both your goals and your current fitness level, the following general suggestions are meant to help you zero in on a practice that's right for you. In the following section, you'll find some of the most common styles of yoga grouped into broad categories. Please understand that as with any compartmentalization, the categories represent a simplistic approach to yoga. Virtually any yoga style is complete in and of itself and has a host of tools that can help you benefit from its teachings. In addition, many yoga teachers are versed in more than one style of yoga so that they may blend syntheses of styles in their own work. However, understanding the general thrust of a particular approach to yoga may very well help you to solve the yoga puzzle as you piece together your own private practice.

Piece #3: Pick From the Various Different Styles of Yoga

The various styles of yoga can be grouped into a few broad, general categories. Understanding your needs and fitness level, you can focus your yoga search on one or more of the following general approaches to yoga practice.

Vigorous, Athletic Approaches to Yoga

Having taken into account your yoga goals and your level of fitness, perhaps you've decided you would like to try a yoga practice that's physically demanding. You may be looking for a strenuous approach to the physical postures of yoga that strengthens your muscles, while also working out your heart. Maybe you feel that you have to sweat to be your own ideal yogi. If that's the case, then you might want to investigate the following styles of yoga: Ashtanga Yoga (vigorous flowing yoga); Iyengar Yoga (physically demanding in its precision); Bikram Yoga (performed in superheated studios); Jivamukti Yoga (physically demanding, eclectic urban yoga); kundalini yoga (challenging both physically and psychoenergetically); and ISHTA Yoga, Power Yoga, Vinyasa Yoga, or White Lotus Yoga (all drawing in varying degrees of Ashtanga Yoga).

Yoga for General Stress-Reduction and Health

After taking stock of your yoga needs, maybe you realize you don't have to huff and puff to feel like you're a real man doing real yoga. Maybe a more relaxing style of yoga that will help you strengthen and stretch more gently is what you're looking for. Then you might want to consider one of the following styles of yoga. Practicing one of the foundational approaches to yoga may be right for you: You can select from yoga taught by Ananda Yoga, the Himalayan Institute, Integral Yoga, Sivananda Yoga, or, for a more contemporary adaptation, Kripalu Yoga. You might also wish to investigate Gary Krafstow's Viniyoga, which can help you fine-tune your practice to wherever you may be in your life's journey.

Yoga for the Perfect Pose

If you're interested in perfecting your yoga poses to reach that idealized perfect alignment, then the premier method of yoga for you may well be Iyengar Yoga. Anusara Yoga and Viniyoga might also interest you. Finally, many teachers who are trained in the Ashtanga Yoga tradition and its derivative styles can help you improve your alignment in postures. If you have a double goal of practicing a demanding style of yoga while also improving your yoga alignment, you may want to investigate Ashtanga Yoga, ISHTA Yoga, Power Yoga, Vinyasa Yoga, and White Lotus Yoga.

Yoga as Therapy

Perhaps you're coming to yoga out of a specific need to help relieve a particular problem or problems—physical, mental, or emotional. Then you'll be pleased to know that there are styles of yoga that can help you achieve this goal. Iyengar Yoga has developed an entire approach to the practice of yoga that draws heavily on the use of props to help you deal with physical limitations and challenges (and who among us doesn't have some limitations?). Integrative Yoga Therapy has trained many teachers specifically to assist people with health problems. Kundalini yoga may help you to connect to core emotional and mental issues. Phoenix Rising Yoga Therapy uses assisted postures and talk therapy to help you not only physically, but also mentally and emotionally. Hidden Language of Hatha Yoga tries to help you connect with the hidden meaning and currents of energy underlying the physical postures of hatha yoga.

Yoga as a Spiritual Quest

Perhaps the yoga practice that's right for you doesn't involve a lot of physical exertion using the traditional postures of hatha yoga. Maybe you're really interested in exploring yoga's rich spiritual tradition and connecting with your inner self through the mind. Then you might want to consider other ways of custom-tailoring a yoga program to suit your needs. Many of the major yoga institutes detailed in the chapters on hatha yoga offer courses in meditation, study of the major spiritual texts that form the basis for yoga, or yogic breathing techniques that can help you to connect to your inner being. Chief among these are the Himalayan Institute, Integral Yoga, Kripalu Yoga, and Sivananda Yoga. You may also want to explore tantric yoga, which uses rituals, such as mantra recitation, and ceremonies to help you connect to the divinity within. You may want to explore karma yoga, the path of self-discovery through service to others. Or you may be an independent type, wishing to read and practice yoga on your own in your own way. In that case, you may want to consult some of the books on yoga in the Bibliography of this book, or visit your local library or bookstore and choose the resource that speaks to your inner knowing.

Piece #4: Discipline and Balance

Once you've given thought to your yoga needs and pieced together a yoga practice that's right for you, try to be as disciplined about your approach to practice as possible. No matter which approach to yoga you decide to follow, remember: Yoga is not a "quick fix." Its benefits are cumulative, and may seem subtle, especially when you first begin to practice it.

Allow yourself the time to practice yoga regularly for awhile before you judge its effects. All too often, men begin a practice of yoga by taking a course or two, and then abandon the practice because they don't feel or see immediate results.

If you're just beginning your practice, try to approach yoga with an open body, mind, and heart. Suspend your judgment and give yoga the benefit of the doubt. Commit to practicing yoga for at least four to six weeks, and see what effect it has on your life. In practicing yoga, it's very beneficial to be regular and disciplined. Ideally, try to practice yoga at least two to three times a week for an hour or so at a time. If that doesn't work for you, then try to practice as often as fits into your schedule for as long as you are able. But do try to be regular and disciplined to reap the greatest rewards from your yoga practice.

In crafting a yoga practice that's right for you, also keep in mind the principle of balance. As one of my teachers advised me: "If you're in a hurry, slow down. If you're going slowly, speed up!" You may want to explore styles of yoga that counterbalance your predominant character and personality traits. If you're a "Type A" overachiever, you may find yourself naturally drawn to a vigorous style of yoga such as Ashtanga Yoga. But then again, you may benefit from a relaxing style of yoga that will help to restore and renew you. If you're a sedentary man, you may want to include some classes in a vigorous style of yoga to get the physical benefits of the practice. And no matter where you are in your life and what style of yoga you are drawn to, you can always mix and match styles to create your own eclectic yoga practice.

And remember to listen always to your body and your breath: They are your own best teachers.

CHAPTER NOTES

Epigraph

1. Winthrop Sargeant, trans., *Bhagavad Gita* (Albany, N.Y.: SUNY, 1994), 135.

Getting Started

1. T.K.V. Desikachar, *The Heart of Yoga* (Rochester, Vt.: Inner Traditions, 1995), 7.

Introduction

1. Sachindra Kumar Majumdar, *Introduction to Yoga Principles and Practices* (New Hyde Park, N.Y.: University Books, 1966), 30.
2. For information on details of principal yoga texts, as well as English translations of Sanskrit names, both here and throughout *Yoga for Men*, I am deeply indebted to the resource information presented in Georg Feuerstein, Ph.D., *The Shambhala Encyclopedia of Yoga* (Boston, Mass.: Shambhala, 1997).
3. Juan Mascaro, trans., *The Bhagavad Gita* (Baltimore, Md.: Penguin Books, 1962), 9.

Chapter 1: The Tree of Yoga

1. B.K.S. Iyengar, *The Tree of Yoga* (Boston: Shambhala, 1988), 77.
2. Swami Rama, *Choosing a Path* (Honesdale, Pa.: Himalayan Institute, 1982), 21.

Part II: Hatha Yoga

1. Feuerstein, op. cit., 121–122.

Chapter 2: Himalayan Institute

1. *Himalayan Institute Quarterly Guide to Programs,* Spring 1998, 19.
2. *Himalayan Institute In Memoriam Program,* Spring 1997, 2.
3. *Yoga International's 1998 Guide to Yoga Teachers and Classes,* 42.
4. *Himalayan Institute Quarterly Guide to Programs,* Spring 1998, 20.

Chapter 4: Iyengar Yoga

1. Iyengar, op. cit., 12.
2. Ibid, 156–157.
3. Ibid, 27.
4. "A Pictorial Biography of Yogacharya B.K.S. Iyengar" at *www.bksiyengar.com.*
5. Iyengar, op. cit., 7–9.
6. Ibid, p. 33.

Chapter 5: Sivananda Yoga

1. Sivananda Yoga Vedanta Center, Winter/Spring 2003 Catalog.
2. *www.sivananda.org.*
3. Ibid.

Chapter 6: Ashtanga Yoga

1. Bernard Bouanchaud, (Rosemary Desneux, trans.), *The Essence of Yoga: Reflections on the Yoga Sutras of Patanjali* (Portland, Oreg.: Rudra Press, 1997), 108–109.
2. Beryl Bender Birch, *Power Yoga* (New York: Fireside, 1995), 20.
3. Fernando Pagés Ruiz, "Krishnamacharya's Legacy," *Yoga Journal,* May/June 2001 (available online at *www.yogajournal.com*).
4. Anne Cushman, "Power Yoga," *Yoga Journal,* January/February 1995 (available online at *www.yogajournal.com*).
5. Ibid.

Chapter 7: Kundalini Yoga

1. Gopi Krishna, *Kundalini: The Evolutionary Energy in Man* (Boston: Shambhala, 1985), 12–13.
2. Shakti Parwha Kaur Khalsa, *Kundalini Yoga: The Flow of Eternal Power* (New York: Perigee, 1996), 48.
3. Feuerstein, op. cit., 346–347.
4. B.K.S. Iyengar, *Light on Pranayama: The Yogic Art of Breathing* (New York: Crossroad, 1997), 36.
5. Swami Rama, et al., *Science of Breath: A Practical Guide* (Honesdale, Pa.: Himalayan Institute, 1979), 77.

6. For more on the chakras, including other variant English translations of their names and the many interesting associations to each chakra, see Harish Johari's *Chakras: Energy Centers of Transformation* (Rochester, Vt.: Destiny Books, 1987).

Chapter 8: Kripalu Yoga

1. *The Kripalu Experience*, n.d. *The Kripalu Experience* is a quarterly program catalog of the Kripalu Center.

Chapter 9: Phoenix Rising Yoga Therapy

1. Michael Lee, *Phoenix Rising Yoga Therapy* (Deerfield Beach, Fla.: Health Communications, Inc., 1997), 6, 29.

2. Daniel J. Wiener, *Beyond Talk Therapy* (Washington, D.C.: American Psychological Association, 1999), 208–209.

Chapter 10: Endless Yoga

1. Majumdar, op. cit., 49.

2. Paramahansa Yogananda, *Autobiography of a Yogi* (Los Angeles, Calif.: Self-Realization Fellowship, 1946), Chapter 37.

Chapter 11: Yoga for the Phases of a Man's Life

1. T.K.V. Desikachar, op. cit., 79.

2. Ruiz, op. cit.

3. For an interesting article profiling individual practitioners of yoga at different ages, see Donna Raskin, "As Time Goes By," *Yoga Journal*, December 2001.

4. Patricia Leigh Brown, "Latest Way to Cut Grade School Stress: Yoga," *The New York Times*, March 24, 2002.

5. Adam Skolnick, "Seeds of Change: Yoga for Troubled Youth" available online at *www.yimag.org*, 2000.

6. Quoted in Georg Feuerstein, trans. and ed., *Teachings of Yoga* (Boston: Shambhala, 1997), 4.

7. Majumdar, op cit., 34.

8. Quoted in Pandit Rajmani Tigunait, Ph.D. *At the Eleventh Hour: The Biography of Swami Rama*, (Honesdale, Pa.: Himalayan Institute Press, 2001), 359.

9. Statistics from the Centers for Disease Control and Prevention, quoted in Maggie Fox, "Healthy Older Americans," a Reuters' news release dated September 12, 2002.

10. For a comprehensive presentation of yoga for mature practitioners, including designing a yoga practice, see Suza Francina, *The New Yoga for People Over 50* (Deerfield Beach, Fla.: Health Communications, 1997).

11. Ibid.

12. Gary Kraftsow, as quoted at *www.viniyoga.com*.

Chapter 12: Yoga for Athletics and Sports

1. Aladar Kogler, Ph.D. *Yoga for Athletes: Secrets of an Olympic Coach* (St. Paul, Minn.: Llewellyn, 1999), xix.
2. For a whimsical and informative first-hand account of one "outsider's" foray into yoga territory, see Tim Cahill, "Yoga Kicked My Butt," *Yoga Journal* (September/October 2000).
3. Gilles Toucas, "Richard Gere, un Homme Engagé," *Santé Fitness* 63 (April 2002): 23.
4. Dimity McDowell, "Yoga for Baseball," *Yoga Journal* (July/August 2000).
5. Joni Hyde, "Stretching for Results" (July 31, 2002) available at *www.yoga.com*.
6. Quoted in McDowell, op. cit.
7. Quoted in Dimity McDowell, "Yoga for Kickboxing," *Yoga Journal* (September/October 2000).

Chapter 13: Yoga for Men's Health

1. Tigunait, Ph.D., op. cit., 354.
2. Joni Hyde, "The Low Down on Low Back Pain" at *www.yoga.com* (July 311, 2002).
3. Pam Germain, "Posture Perfect" at *www.yoga.com* (August 2, 2002).
4. *www.prostateaction.org* (the Website of Prostate Action, Inc.).
5. Claudia Kalb, et al., "Coping with Anxiety," *Newsweek*, 24 February 2003.
6. Kathryn Black, "Yoga under the Microscope" at *www.yogajournal.com*.
7. Ibid. And Alice Lesch Kelly, "Rest for the Weary" at *www.yogajournal.com*.
8. Weiner, op. cit., 217.

Chapter 14: Yoga and a Man's Sex Life

1. Swami Rama, *Choosing a Path*, 56.
2. Todd Jones, "The Truth about Tantra," *Yoga Journal* (January/February 2000).
3. Ibid.
4. Ibid.
5. Pala Copeland and Al Link, *Soul Sex: Tantra for Two* (Franklin Lakes, N.J.: Career Press, 2003), 147. See pages 146–149 for additional information and instructions on PC exercises.
6. David Strovny, "Kegel Exercises for Men" at *www.AskMen.com*.
7. Loraine Despres, "Yoga's Bad Boy: Bikram Choudhury," *Yoga Journal* (March/April 2000).
8. Tigunait, Ph.D., op cit., 235.

Part V: The Yoga Lifestyle

1. Swami Venkatesananda, The Concise Yoga Vasistha (Albany, N.Y.: State University of New York Press, 1984), 212-222.

Chapter 16: The Yoga Lifestyle

1. Quoted on the *www.whitelotus.org* home page.
2. Swami Rama, *Choosing a Path*, 192.
3. For further information on yogic reasons for being a vegetarian, see Sivananda Yoga Vedanta Center's *Yoga Mind & Body* (New York: DK Publishing, 1996), 126–127.
4. Ibid, 128–129.
5. Ibid, 150–151.
6. Desikachar, op. cit., 22.
7. Swami Rama, *Choosing a Path*, 17.
8. Swami Sivananda, *Sadhana* (Tehri-Garhwal, India: Divine Life Society Publications, 1998), 458–461. Edited and abridged, with parenthetical translations added to aid understanding.

Afterword: The Yoga Puzzle

1. Lee, op. cit., 150.
2. For readers interested in taking a tongue-in-cheek, yet informative, quiz to find out which style of yoga suits you best, see Todd Jones's, "Are You a Sweat-Hog or a Swami?" available at *www.yogajournal.com*. Also of interest at the same Website is Jennifer Cook, "Not All Yoga Is Created Equal."

Postscript

1. Quoted in Sandra Anderson and Rolf Sovik, Psy.D., *Yoga: Mastering the Basics* (Honesdale, Pa.: Himalayan Institute Press, 2000), "Dedication."

BIBLIOGRAPHY

Ajaya, Swami, Ph.D. *Yoga Psychology: A Practical Guide to Meditation.* Honesdale, Pa.: Himalayan Institute Press, 1976.

Anderson, Bob. *Stretching for Everyday Fitness and for Running, Tennis, Racquetball, Cycling, Swimming, Golf, and Other Sports.* Bolinas, Calif.: Shelter Publications, 1980.

Anderson, Sandra, and Rolf Sovik, Psy.D. *Yoga: Mastering the Basics.* Honesdale, Pa.: Himalayan Institute Press, 2000.

Arya, Pandit Usharbudh, D.Litt. *Superconscious Meditation.* Honesdale, Pa.: Himalayan Institute Press, 1978.

Ballentine, Rudolph M., M.D. ed. *The Theory and Practice of Meditation,* 2nd ed. Honesdale, Pa.: Himalayan Institute Press, 1986.

Benson, Herbert, M.D. *The Relaxation Response.* New York: William Morrow, 1975.

Blumenfeld, Larry, ed. *The Big Book of Relaxation: Simple Techniques to Control the Excess Stress in Your Life.* Roslyn, N.Y.: The Relaxation Company, 1994.

Bouanchaud, Bernard. *The Essence of Yoga: Reflections on the Yoga Sutras of Patanjali.* Translated by Rosemary Desneux. Portland, Oreg.: Rudra Press, 1997.

Desikachar, T.K.V. *The Heart of Yoga: Developing a Personal Practice.* Rochester, Vt.: Inner Traditions International, 1999.

Easwaran, Eknath. *Meditation: A Simple 8-Point Program for Translating Spiritual Ideals into Daily Life,* 2nd ed. Tomales, Calif.: Niligri Press, 1991.

Feuerstein, Georg, Ph.D. *The Shambhala Guide to Yoga: An Essential Introduction to the Principles and Practice of an Ancient Tradition.* Boston: Shambhala, 1996.

————. *The Shambhala Encyclopedia of Yoga.* Boston: Shambhala, 1997.

————. trans. and ed. *Teachings of Yoga*. Boston: Shambhala, 1997.

————, and Stephan Bodian, with the staff of *Yoga Journal*, eds., *Living Yoga: A Comprehensive Guide for Daily Life*. New York: Jeremy P. Tarcher, 1993.

————, and Jeanine Miller. *The Essence of Yoga: Essays on the Development of Yogic Philosophy from the Vedas to Modern Times*. Rochester, Vt.: Inner Traditions International, 1998.

————, and Larry Payne, Ph.D. *Yoga for Dummies: A Reference for the Rest of Us*. Foster City, Calif.: IDG Books Worldwide, 1999.

Iyengar, B.K.S. *Light on Pranayama: The Yogic Art of Breathing*. New York: Crossroad, 1997.

————. *The Tree of Yoga*. Boston: Shambhala, 1988.

————. *Yoga: The Path to Holistic Health*. New York: Dorling Kindersley, 2001.

Johari, Harish. *Chakras: Energy Centers of Transformation*. Rochester, Vt.: Destiny Books, 1987.

Kabat-Zinn, Jon, Ph.D. *Full Catastrophe Living: Using the Wisdom of Your Body and Mind to Face Stress, Pain, and Illness*. New York: Delta, 1990.

Kilham, Christopher S. *The Five Tibetans: Five Dynamic Exercises for Health, Energy, and Personal Power*. Rochester, Vt.: Healing Arts Press, 1994.

Klein, Jean. *La Joie sans Objet*. Paris: Mercure de France, 1977.

————. *Qui Suis-je? La quête sacrée*. Paris: Albin Michel, 1989.

Krishna, Gopi. *Kundalini: The Evolutionary Energy in Man*. Boston: Shambhala, 1985.

Lasater, Judith, Ph.D., P.T. *Relax & Renew: Restful Yoga for Stressful Times*. Berkeley, Calif.: Rodmell Press, 1995.

Lee, Michael. *Phoenix Rising Yoga Therapy: A Bridge from Body to Soul*. Deerfield Beach, Fla.: Health Communications, 1997.

Majumdar, Sachindra Kumar. *Introduction to Yoga Principles and Practices*. New Hyde Park, N.Y.: University Books, 1965.

Mohan, A.G. *Yoga for Body, Breath, and Mind: A Guide to Personal Reintegration*. Boston: Shambhala, 2002.

Muktananda, Swami. *Play of Consciousness*. South Fallsburg, N.Y.: SYDA Foundation, 2000.

Myers, Esther. *Yoga and You: Energizing and Relaxing Yoga for New and Experienced Students*. Boston: Shambhala, 1997.

Nuernberger, Phil, Ph.D. *Freedom from Stress: A Holistic Approach*. Honesdale, Pa.: Himalayan Institute Press, 1981.

Prakash, Prem. *The Yoga of Spiritual Devotion: A Modern Translation of the Narada Bhakti Sutras*. Rochester, Vt.: Inner Traditions International, 1998.

Rama, Sri Swami. *Choosing a Path*. Honesdale, Pa.: Himalayan Institute Press, 1982.

————. *Living with the Himalayan Masters: Spiritual Experiences of Swami Rama*. Honesdale, Pa.: Himalayan Institute Press, 1978.

————, and Swami Ajaya. *Creative Use of Emotion*. Honesdale, Pa.: Himalayan Institute Press, 1976.

Rhada, Swami Sivananda. *Hatha Yoga: The Hidden Language.* Spokane, Wash.: Timeless Books, 1995.

———. *Kundalini Yoga for the West: A Foundation for Character Building, Courage and Awareness.* Spokane, Wash.: Timeless Books, 1993.

Rosen, Richard. *The Yoga of Breath: A Step-by-Step Guide to Pranayama.* Boston: Shambhala, 2002.

Schatz, Mary Pullig, M.D. *Back Care Basics: A Doctor's Gentle Yoga Program for Back and Neck Pain Relief.* Berkeley, Calif.: Rodmell Press, 1992.

Sivananda Yoga Vedanta Center. *Yoga Mind & Body.* New York: Dorling Kindersley, 1996.

Shivapremananda, Swami. *Yoga for Stress Relief: A Simple and Unique Three-Month Program for De-Stressing and Stress Prevention.* New York: Random House, 1997.

Tigunait, Pandit Rajmani, Ph.D. *At the Eleventh Hour: The Biography of Swami Rama.* Honesdale, Pa.: Himalayan Institute Press, 2001.

Venkatesananda, Swami. *The Concise Yoga Vasistha.* Albany, N.Y.: State University of New York Press, 1984.

Vishnu-devananda, Swami. *The Complete Illustrated Book of Yoga.* New York: Bell Publishing Company, Inc., 1960.

Yogananda, Paramahansa. *Autobiography of a Yogi,* 12th ed. Los Angeles: Self-Realization Fellowship, 1993.

Postscript

As you embark on your own journey of yoga, may you be inspired by the verses of the Sanskrit *Asato Ma* prayer:

Lead me from the unreal to the real

Lead me from darkness to light

Lead me from mortality to immortality

OM shantih shantih shantih

OM peace peace peace.[1]

INDEX

About the Author

Thomas Claire is a writer, body/mind practitioner, and personal development facilitator. He is the author of the critically acclaimed guide to massage and bodywork, *Bodywork: What Type of Massage to Get—and How to Make the Most of It* (William Morrow, 1995).

Thomas is an assistant professor at Queensborough Community College City University of New York. He teaches Eastern anatomy and bodywork in the Healing Arts division in an innovative program that he helped design and implement. He lives and works in New York City.

Thomas has been practicing yoga for more than 30 years. His goal is to help each individual connect with his or her own inner guru by presenting tools for inner transformation drawn from a wide range of traditions in as simple and clear a manner as possible. Thomas facilitates classes, workshops, and intensive private sessions in personal transformation practices around the world.

For further information on his work, you can visit him at his Website: *www.thomasclaire.com.*

You can also write to him at:

Thomas Claire

c/o Clairefontaine, Inc.

P.O. Box 1040

Grand Central Station

New York, NY 10163-1040

Author's Special Appreciation

The author would like to extend my special appreciation to Thomas Amador, who photographed the illustrations in *Yoga for Men*. Through his gifted eye, he helped bring the words in this book to life; through his peaceful being, he brought out the best in everyone. Tom lives in New York City, where he works as a freelance photographer, a Thai massage therapist, and a yoga instructor. He is an avid cyclist. His photography has been featured in prominent New York City gallery exhibitions.